ENDOCRINOLOGY

made ridiculously simple

Stephen Goldberg, MD
Professor Emeritus
University of Miami
Miller School of Medicine
Miami, Florida

MEDMASTER

ISBN #978-1-962445-00-9
eISBN 9781962445016

Made in the United States of America

Published by Medmaster, Inc.
3389 Sheridan St., #243
Hollywood, FL 33021

Cover design by Matteo Farinella
Inside Illustrations by Jordan Collver and Isabel Loureiro

Contents

Preface

Endocrinology encompasses numerous interrelated diseases. It is easy to get lost in its complexity. This book is directed toward the medical, nursing, and PA student as well as the general practitioner, who would like a brief overview of the key clinical aspects of endocrinology, with understanding, rather than rote memorization.

This is not a reference book; there are other excellent sources with detailed instructions in the step-by-step quantitative management of complex endocrine problems. Rather, this book aims to provide an overall understanding of clinical endocrinology with its interweaving associations of hormones, the mechanisms of hormone actions, the diseases that may arise from oversecretion or undersecretion, and the logic behind the diagnosis and treatment of the most common endocrine conditions.

I thank Samuel Sugar, MD, FACP, as well as Michael A. Chizner, MD, Clinical Professor of Medicine, University of Miami Miller School of Medicine, Director of Medical Education, Simulation, Continuing Medical Education and Clinical Innovation, Broward Health, and author of *Clinical Cardiology Made Ridiculously Simple* for their reviews and helpful comments. I am also indebted to Phyllis Goldenberg for her superb proofreading and advice.

Stephen Goldberg, MD

Chapter 1 **Introduction**

Endocrinology is the study of **hormones**, their functions in health and disease, and the diagnosis and treatment of their disorders. Hormones are chemical messengers that enter the bloodstream and affect the function of cells distant from the site of secretion. They influence cell behavior, including the breakdown of nutrients to produce energy, the synthesis of molecules necessary for cellular function, and the regulation of various physiological activities.

The term **endocrine** differs from **exocrine**, **paracrine**, and **autocrine**.

- **Exocrine glands** secrete their chemicals into a *duct*, e.g., sweat, tears, milk, saliva, digestive enzymes, rather than into the bloodstream.
- **Paracrine** signaling (**Fig. 1-1**) is molecular communication between *nearby* cells within a tissue, e.g., cytokines released by immune cells; cell release of growth factors that aid local wound healing and clotting; neurotransmitters that convey nerve signals.
- **Autocrine** signaling (**Fig. 1-1**) occurs when a cell secretes a chemical that binds to the cell's *own* receptors, causing changes within that cell, such as T-cell activation by IL-2, which acts on the same T-cell to promote its proliferation.

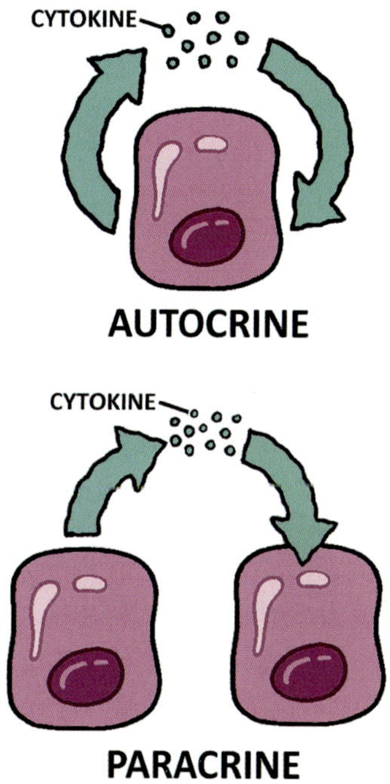

Fig. 1-1. Autocrine and Paracrine Signaling. (From Goldberg, S. Clinical Physiology Made Ridiculously Simple. Medmaster.)

Hormones can have different types of structure. Some are *proteins* or *peptides* (composed of amino acids), e.g., insulin, growth hormone, glucagon, parathyroid hormone, prolactin, follicle-stimulating hormone. Others are *steroids* (derived from cholesterol), e.g., cortisol, aldosterone, testosterone, and estrogen. Others are *amines* ("monoamine hormones"), derived from the amino acid tyrosine (epinephrine, norepinephrine, dopamine, thyroid hormone) or tryptophan (serotonin, melatonin).

Hormones differ from **enzymes**. Enzymes are catalysts, generally proteins (although some are RNA molecules), which speed up chemical reactions without being changed. They usually act locally, either within the cell or nearby. Hormones, though, do not speed up chemical reactions. They are chemical messengers that are produced by endocrine glands and travel in the bloodstream to target tissues to activate or deactivate specific chemical pathways, sometimes altering gene expression.

Back-and-forth hormonal **feedback** signaling is important throughout the body to ensure that body metabolism stays balanced (**homeostasis**) and the organs and tissues work as a unified and healthy whole, rather than as an anarchy of isolated parts. For instance, the pituitary gland secretes hormones that activate other glands in various parts of the body. Those glands in turn, release hormones that, as part of their effect, feed back to the pituitary and modify the amount of its secretion, so that it is not too much or too little (**Figs. 1-2** and **1-3**).

Perhaps the simplest example of negative feedback is in the basic chemical reaction

$$A + B \rightarrow C$$

As the concentration of molecule C increases, it tends to push back and reduce the reaction of A + B from going to the right.

Feedback regulation occurs throughout the endocrine system but in a more complex way. For instance, in **Figure 1-3** the hypothalamus stimulates the pituitary gland to produce thyroid-stimulating hormone (TSH), which stimulates the thyroid gland to produce thyroid hormone (T4 and T3). Thyroid hormone feeds back to the hypothalamus and pituitary gland to reduce their secretion (negative feedback). This ensures that the level of thyroid hormone in the body remains balanced. Negative feedback (and sometimes positive feedback) is common throughout the endocrine system.

Hormonal actions in endocrinology are very much interconnected. Endocrinology resembles a giant spider web, or system of interlocking rivers, in which motion at any point can cause changes throughout the system.

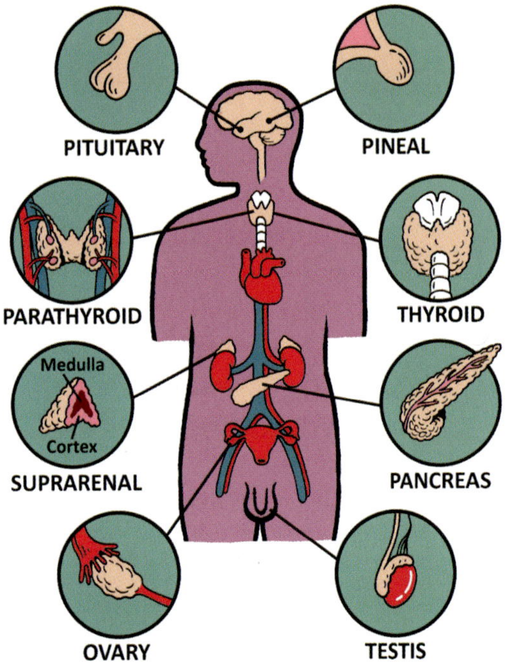

Fig. 1-2. The main endocrine glands. (From Goldberg, S. Clinical Physiology Made Ridiculously Simple. Medmaster.)

The Hormones

Figure 1-4 lists the main hormones of the body and their general functions.

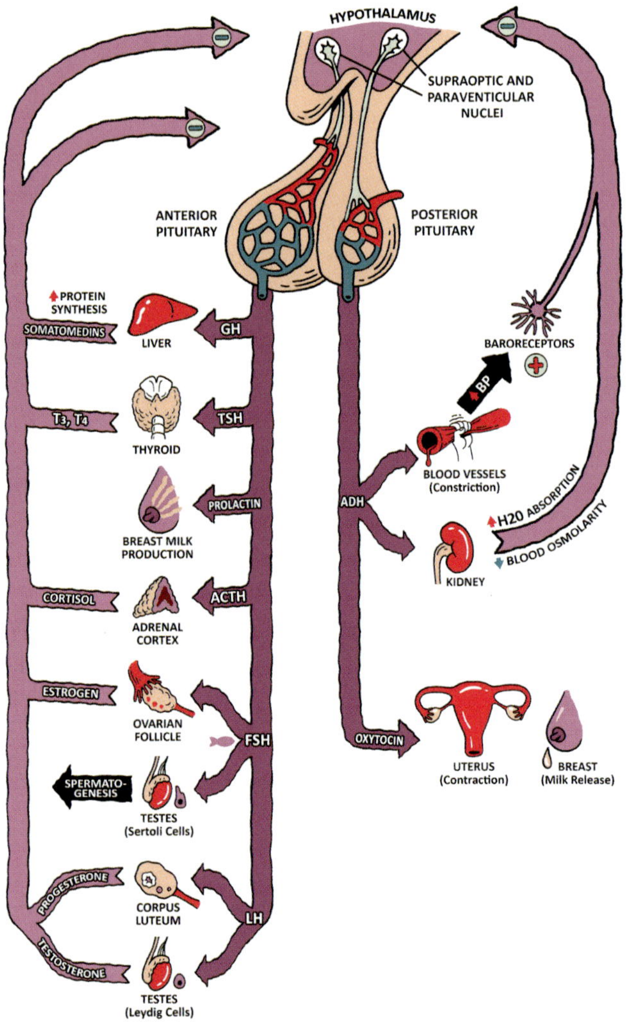

Fig. 1-3. The pituitary gland receives mainly negative feedback from the glands that it stimulates, thus preventing pituitary oversecretion or undersecretion. (From Goldberg, S. Clinical Physiology Made Ridiculously Simple. Medmaster.)

FIGURE 1-4. THE MAJOR HORMONES OF THE BODY	
Organ	**Hormones and Their Main Functions**
Pancreas	• **Insulin** decreases blood glucose levels by moving glucose from the bloodstream into cells and promoting its storage and utilization for energy. • **Glucagon** *increases* blood glucose, the opposite of insulin, by promoting glucose production and its release into the bloodstream when glucose is low. • **Somatostatin** inhibits hormone secretion, including insulin, glucagon, gastrointestinal hormones, growth hormone and others, to help keep hormone balance within a narrow range. • **Pancreatic polypeptide** inhibits the secretion of pancreatic enzymes and insulin and promotes glucagon release; decreases appetite after a meal; modulates the pH and motility of the digestive system.
Thyroid gland	• **T4 (thyroxine)** and **T3 (triiodothyronine)**, together called **thyroid hormone**, stimulate metabolism, growth, and development in cells throughout the body. • **Calcitonin** decreases blood calcium levels, the opposite of parathyroid hormone, by inhibiting bone breakdown and promoting calcium excretion by the kidneys.
Parathyroid gland	• **Parathyroid Hormone (PTH)** increases calcium levels in the blood by promoting calcium release from bone (*bone resorption*) and enhancing calcium reabsorption from the kidneys. PTH also stimulates production of active vitamin D, which promotes intestinal absorption and renal reabsorption of calcium.
Adrenal gland	• **Cortisol**, the "stress hormone," helps the body respond to stress by increasing blood glucose levels for energy, suppressing the immune system so that is not overactive, increasing blood pressure, and helping maintain a stable mood. • **Aldosterone** increases blood pressure and blood fluid volume and helps regulate electrolyte balance by promoting sodium and water reabsorption and potassium excretion in the kidneys. • **DHEA (dehydroepiandrosterone)** is an androgenic precursor hormone, which can be converted in the periphery into testosterone and, to a lesser extent, estrogens. • **Epinephrine and Norepinephrine** increase heart rate, blood pressure, and energy availability to prepare for the "fight-or-flight" response.
Ovary	• **Estradiol, Estriol,** and **Estrone** are forms of estrogen that play key roles in the development and maintenance of female reproductive tissues, secondary female sexual characteristics, and regulation of the menstrual cycle. • **Progesterone** helps prepare and maintain the uterus for pregnancy, supports embryo implantation, and helps regulate the menstrual cycle.
Testis	• **Testosterone** promotes the development and maintenance of male reproductive tissues and secondary male sexual characteristics, sperm production, libido, muscle mass, and overall sexual and reproductive function in males.
Pituitary gland	• **Adrenocorticotropic Hormone (ACTH; corticotropin)** stimulates the adrenal gland to produce and release cortisol and androgens, and, to a minimal degree, aldosterone. • **Thyroid-stimulating Hormone (TSH)** stimulates the thyroid gland to produce and release thyroid hormones T3 and T4. • **Growth Hormone (GH; somatotropin)** stimulates growth, cell reproduction, and regeneration in various tissues and organs. • **Follicle-stimulating Hormone (FSH)** stimulates the growth and development of ovarian follicles in females and promotes sperm production in males. • **Luteinizing Hormone (LH)**, in females, stimulates estrogen and progesterone production in the ovary as well as ovulation, and promotes the production of testosterone in males. • **Prolactin** stimulates breast development during pregnancy and milk production following childbirth and supports maternal nurturing behaviors.

(*Continued*)

FIGURE 1-4. THE MAJOR HORMONES OF THE BODY (CONTINUED)	
Organ	**Hormones and Their Main Functions**
Hypothalamus	• **Oxytocin** promotes milk ejection during breastfeeding, stimulates uterine contractions during childbirth, and facilitates social bonding between individuals. • **Antidiuretic Hormone (ADH; vasopressin)** increases water reabsorption in the kidney to maintain body fluids and increases blood pressure when needed by vasoconstriction. • **Gonadotropin-releasing Hormone (GnRH)** stimulates the release of follicle-stimulating hormone (FSH) and luteinizing hormone (LH) from the anterior pituitary gland. • **Thyrotropin-releasing Hormone (TRH)** stimulates the secretion of thyroid-stimulating hormone (TSH) from the anterior pituitary. TSH, in turn, stimulates the thyroid gland to produce thyroid hormone. • **Corticotropin-releasing Hormone (CRH)** stimulates the release of adrenocorticotropic hormone (ACTH) from the anterior pituitary. ACTH then triggers the release of cortisol and DHEA (dehydroepiandrosterone) from the adrenal glands. • **Growth Hormone-releasing Hormone (GHRH)** stimulates the secretion of growth hormone (GH) from the anterior pituitary. • **Growth Hormone-inhibiting Hormone (GHIH; somatostatin)** inhibits the secretion of growth hormone (GH) as well as thyroid-stimulating hormone (TSH) and ACTH from the anterior pituitary. • **Prolactin-inhibiting Hormone (dopamine)** inhibits the secretion of prolactin and TSH from the anterior pituitary.
Pineal gland	• **Melatonin** promotes the onset of sleep.
Thymus	• **Thymosin** helps regulate the development and maturation of T-cells.
Heart	• **Atrial Natriuretic Peptide (ANP)** and **B-type Natriuretic Peptide (BNP)** decrease blood pressure by vasodilation and promote excretion of sodium and water in the urine, thus counteracting hypertension and fluid retention.
Lungs	• The lungs produce the enzyme **Angiotensin-converting Enzyme (ACE).** ACE converts the hormone angiotensin I to angiotensin II, which constricts blood vessels, promotes the release of aldosterone by the adrenal gland and vasopressin (ADH) by the hypothalamus, and promotes sodium and water reabsorption in the kidney, all of which help increase and maintain blood pressure and fluid balance in the body.
Kidneys	• **Renin** activates the renin-angiotensin-aldosterone system, leading, in a chain of reactions, to the production of angiotensin II, which helps increase and maintain blood pressure and fluid balance. • **Erythropoietin** stimulates the production of red blood cells (*erythropoiesis*) in the bone marrow to maintain adequate oxygen-carrying capacity in the blood, • **Vitamin D** promotes absorption of calcium and phosphate from the intestines and kidneys, and deposition of calcium and phosphorus in the bones. (It can have the opposite effect on bone, removing calcium from bone when calcium is needed in the blood.) It also supports immune function.
Adipose (fat) tissue	• **Leptin** (the "*satiety hormone*") acts on the hypothalamus to suppress appetite, increase metabolism and maintain weight. It also plays a role in maintaining a normal menstrual cycle and interacting with other hormones. • **Adinopectin** enhances insulin sensitivity, helping to lower blood glucose. It has anti-inflammatory and anti-diabetic effects.
Stomach and intestines	• **Ghrelin** (the "*hunger hormone*") stimulates appetite. • **Gastrin** aids digestion by stimulating gastric acid and enzyme secretion and increasing gastric motility. • **Cholecystokinin** stimulates the contraction of the gallbladder and release of digestive enzymes from the pancreas; it regulates satiety by signaling fullness and reducing appetite. • **Incretin** is a group of hormones that includes **Glucagon-like Peptide-1** (**GLP-1**) and **Glucose-dependent Insulinotropic Peptide** (**GIP**), which stimulate insulin secretion from the pancreas and inhibit the release of glucagon in response to food intake, helping reduce post-meal blood sugar spikes. Incretin also increases the feeling of satiety, reducing food intake by acting on the hypothalamus; incretin also slows down the emptying of the stomach.

(*Continued*)

FIGURE 1-4. THE MAJOR HORMONES OF THE BODY (CONTINUED)	
Organ	**Hormones and Their Main Functions**
Liver	• **Insulin-like Growth Factor 1 (IGF-1; somatomedin C)** promotes growth and development, particularly during childhood and adolescence. Its secretion is stimulated by pituitary growth hormone (GH). • **Thrombopoietin (TPO)** stimulates the production and maturation of platelets in the bone marrow. It plays an important role in regulating blood clotting and platelet levels. • **Angiotensinogen** is involved in the regulation of blood pressure. It is converted by renin into angiotensin I and subsequently, by lung Angiotensin-converting Enzyme (ACE), to angiotensin II. Angiotensin II is a potent vasoconstrictor that also stimulates aldosterone secretion by the adrenal gland and vasopressin (ADH) secretion by the hypothalamus. • **Hepcidin** regulates iron homeostasis. It decreases the absorption and release of iron from the intestine and storage sites, thus influencing overall iron levels in the body and preventing iron overload. • **Sex Hormone-binding Globulin (SHBG)**, while not a hormone, is a protein produced by the liver that binds in the bloodstream to sex hormones such as testosterone and estrogen. It helps regulate the availability and activity of these hormones in the body.
Placenta	• **Human Chorionic Gonadotropin (hCG)** supports pregnancy by promoting the production of progesterone and estrogen. • **Relaxin** relaxes and softens various connective tissues, including ligaments and the cervix, during pregnancy to facilitate childbirth and accommodate fetal growth. • **Human Placental Lactogen (hPL)** contributes to breast changes during pregnancy, including increased sensitivity to prolactin; it increases the breakdown of fats to provide fatty acid energy for the mother, and it contributes to increased insulin resistance in the mother, ensuring more glucose for the fetus.

Endocrine Diagnosis and Treatment

Hormone secretion can be too much or too little, resulting in different endocrine problems. For the healthcare provider to diagnose an endocrine disorder, something about the patient needs to first call attention to the possibility of a hormonal imbalance. It could the symptoms and signs with which the patient presents. In the case of a genetic disease, there may be a whole complex of unique signs and symptoms. The patient's medical and family history, lifestyle, and physical exam may provide the first clues. Or there may be some abnormality in routine blood and urine tests that makes the healthcare provider think there may be an endocrine problem. A single abnormal lab value or physical sign or symptom may be non-specific, but a cluster may point to an endocrine condition that warrants more specialized tests, followed by treatment.

There is a familiar approach to diagnosing endocrine problems:

1. Medical history and physical examination commonly provide important diagnostic information.
2. Bloods tests can measure hormone levels, e.g., thyroid hormones (TSH, T4, T3), reproductive hormones (estrogen, progesterone, testosterone), cortisol, insulin, growth hormone and others, depending on the suspected condition.
3. Urine tests, e.g., a 24-hour urine collection may detect excessive excretion of hormones or their metabolic products.
4. Stimulation and suppression tests. The response of the target organs to particular substances, in comparison with the normal state, helps evaluate whether the glands are functioning normally.
5. Imaging studies, e.g., X-rays, MRI, CT scan, ultrasound, bone scan, or more specialized tests, like PET (Positive Emission Tomography) scans with radioactive tracer substances, are used to visualize and assess the structure and function of specific endocrine organs, such as the thyroid, pituitary, or adrenal glands, or to look for ectopic endocrine tumors.

   CT (Computerized Tomography) scans are excellent for visualizing bones and detecting calcifications. They are relatively fast compared to MRI (Magnetic Resonance Imaging) and useful for patients with difficulty holding still.

However, they do involve radiation exposure, unlike an MRI, and are not as good as an MRI for soft tissue visualization. MRIs, though, can be more expensive, and are contraindicated in patients with metallic implants.
6. Biopsy or fine needle aspiration is used for more definitive histological diagnosis, and to determine whether a mass is benign or malignant.
7. Genetic testing is done where indicated to identify specific gene mutations or chromosomal abnormalities associated with inherited endocrine disorders.

Sometimes, multiple tests are necessary to arrive at a diagnosis, since a single test may not be sensitive or specific enough. For instance, an MRI alone might not be sensitive enough to detect a particularly small endocrine tumor or specific enough to tell whether it is benign or malignant. A hormone level that is adequate for one person may not be for another; or certain hormone levels may have only a short half-life or be cyclic and differ depending on the time of day the blood was drawn or what foods or drugs the patient may have ingested. Therefore, several kinds of diagnostic tests may be needed.

Rather than opting for a shotgun approach and ordering everything, the practitioner, with experience, should be able to select among the tests, prioritizing for testing those diagnoses that are more probable, more serious if missed, and more likely to lead to an effective remedy. Also, the methods of diagnosis and treatment should not be worse than the disease.

In treating an endocrine problem, it is best to address the cause where possible (e.g., surgery to remove an over-secreting tumor; administering a hormone that is deficient; suppressing a hormone that is excessive). When this is not possible, treating the symptoms alone can be most helpful.

All the above approaches can be seen in one form or another in the evaluation and treatment of the endocrine disorders throughout this book.

Chapter 2 **The Pancreas**

The pancreas is both endocrine and exocrine (**Fig. 2-1**). As an exocrine gland, it secretes digestive enzymes into the pancreatic duct and small intestine. As an endocrine gland, the pancreas secretes four main hormones into the bloodstream (**Fig. 2-2**):

- Insulin
- Glucagon
- Somatostatin
- Pancreatic polypeptide

Insulin

The **islets of Langerhans** (**Fig. 2-1**) are clusters of specialized hormone-secreting cells in the pancreas that play a crucial role in regulating blood sugar levels. The islets contain several different types of hormone-secreting cells: Alpha (glucagon), Beta (insulin), Delta (somatostatin), and PP (pancreatic polypeptide) cells.

Beta cells, which make up most of the islet cells, secrete **insulin**. Insulin facilitates the entry of glucose into cells for energy or for storage and lowers blood glucose levels in the process. In liver and muscle cells, glucose is stored as glycogen (**glycogenesis**), a complex carbohydrate. Glucose can also be broken down (**glycolysis**) and stored in fat cells as triglycerides. Or, the glucose can be broken down (**glycolysis**) to acetyl CoA and immediately used for energy in the mitochondrial Krebs cycle, which generates energy-rich ATP molecules (**Figs. 2-3A and 2-3B**).

Glucose, triglycerides, or even proteins can be used as a source of energy, depending on need. In times of plenty, glucose is the main source of energy. In times of starvation, or lack of insulin, the liver at first breaks down glycogen to supply needed glucose (**glycogenolysis**), but since the liver only has enough glycogen stores to last about a day, the fat cells are then called upon to break down their triglycerides to form fatty acids (**lipolysis**), which can be used as fuel by converting to acetyl CoA that enters the mitochondrial Krebs cycle (**Fig. 2-3B**). (Muscle glycogen can also be broken down for energy, but this is more to supply the muscle's own need for glucose, rather than supplying it to the rest of the body.) Glucose can also be formed from non-carbohydrate sources (**gluconeogenesis**), for instance from glycerol derived from triglycerides, or from amino acids derived from protein breakdown, although the body would prefer not to break down its proteins, which have other important functions besides supplying fuel (e.g., as enzymes or structural materials).

Insulin drives glucose into cells for energy and storage. With too much insulin, there may be too little glucose left in the blood for the cells' needs (**hypoglycemia**). With too *little* insulin (**diabetes**), the blood glucose rises (**hyperglycemia**) because the glucose can't get into the cells. Moreover, the cells interpret their lack of glucose as a need for glucose, so the liver breaks down its glycogen (**glycogenolysis**), the fat cells break down their triglycerides (**lipolysis**)

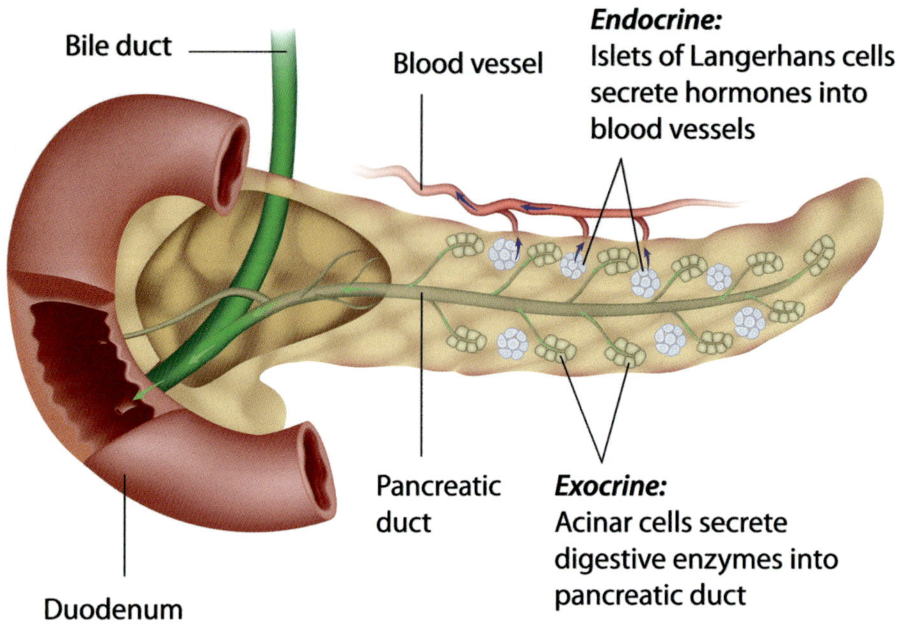

Fig. 2-1. Endocrine and exocrine function of the pancreas.

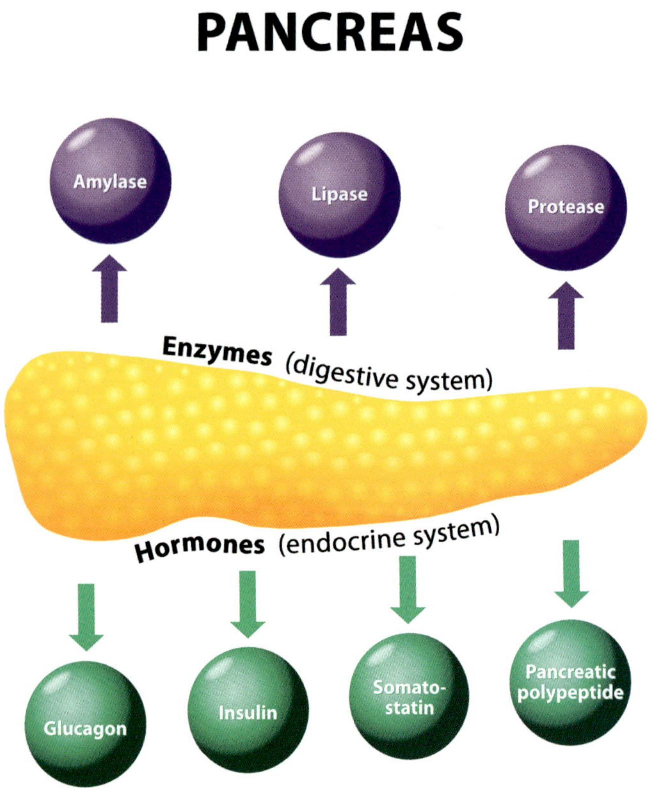

Fig. 2-2. Hormones and enzymes produced by the pancreas.

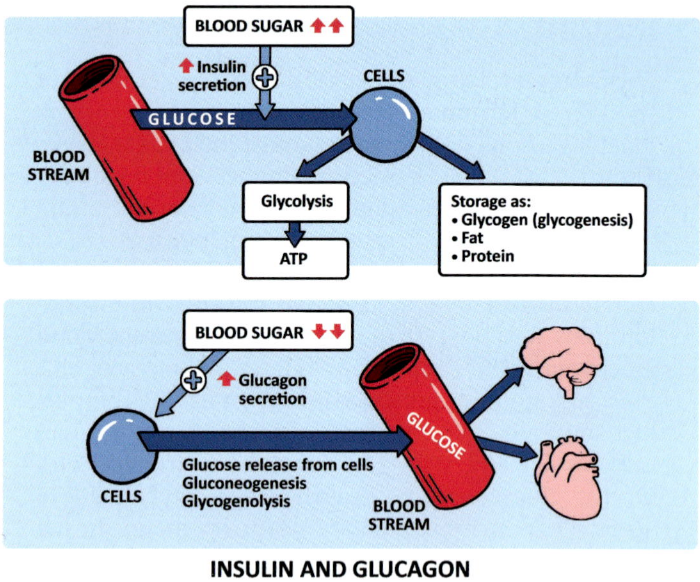

Fig. 2-3A. Insulin vs glucagon.

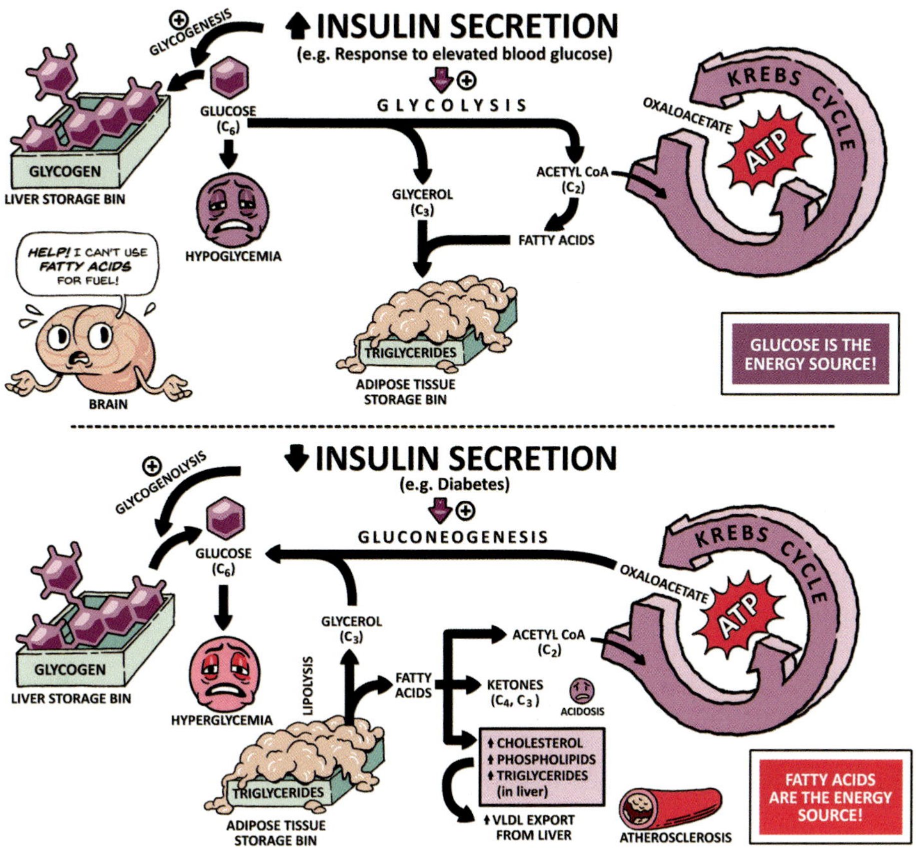

Fig. 2-3B. Effects of insulin on blood glucose. (From Goldberg, S. Clinical Physiology Made Ridiculously Simple. Medmaster.)

and tissue proteins may break down, to form even more blood glucose (**gluconeogenesis**), along with the clinical manifestations of hyperglycemia (**Fig 2-5**).

The brain relies on glucose as its main fuel, since fatty acids do not easily cross the blood-brain barrier (although fatty acids can be converted into ketone fuel for the brain under certain conditions, e.g., starvation, highly ketogenic diets, and insulin deficiency). As extra insurance, brain cells can take up glucose in the absence of insulin.

Alpha cells produce **glucagon**, which has the opposite effect of insulin. Glucagon stimulates the liver to break down glycogen into glucose (**glycogenolysis**) and release it into the bloodstream. This raises blood sugar levels and provides a homeostatic counterbalance to insulin.

Delta cells produce **somatostatin**, which inhibits the secretion of *both* insulin and glucagon, helping in its own way to maintain a proper balance of glucose. Somatostatin is also produced elsewhere in the body (e.g., hypothalamus, GI tract) and is generally inhibitory ("*static*") in nature. Somatostatin from the hypothalamus, where it is also called **Growth Hormone-inhibiting Hormone (GHIH)**, inhibits the release of growth hormone and thyroid-stimulating hormone. In the GI tract, somatostatin inhibits the secretion of gastric acid, pancreatic enzymes, and bile, and slows the movement of food through the digestive tract. It can also inhibit the release of certain neurotransmitters, including dopamine, serotonin, norepinephrine, and acetylcholine. Lest somatostatin be prejudicially judged in a totally negative light, it can also inhibit the growth of certain tumors, particularly those that have receptors for somatostatin. Certain synthetic analogues of somatostatin (e.g., *octreotide* and *lanreotide*) are sometimes used to treat neuroendocrine tumors.

Pancreatic Polypeptide (PP) cells secrete **pancreatic polypeptide**, which primarily inhibits the exocrine function of the pancreas. It suppresses the release of pancreatic enzymes, reduces gallbladder contraction, decreases the secretion of stomach acid, and slows gastric emptying. It may play a role in regulating appetite and food intake, acting as a satiety signal.

All these pancreatic hormones work together to maintain healthy levels of blood glucose.

Diabetes and Hyperglycemia

Diabetes mellitus is a disease of either insulin deficiency or insulin resistance, resulting either way in excess blood sugar (**hyperglycemia**).

Type 1 diabetes is an autoimmune condition with a genetic tendency, in which the immune system mistakenly attacks and destroys the insulin-producing beta cells in the pancreas, resulting in high blood sugar. Potential environmental triggers have also been proposed – viral infections (e.g., coxsackievirus, rotavirus), early childhood exposure to certain foods (e.g., cow's milk, gluten), vitamin D deficiency, gut microbiota disruptions early in life, and a higher incidence in cold climates.

Type 2 diabetes also generates high blood sugar, but by resistance to insulin rather than a lack of it. Type 2 diabetes is probably caused by a combination of genetic factors and lifestyle choices (e.g., poor diet, lack of physical activity, obesity). The concordance rate for type 2 diabetes in monozygotic twins is more than 90%. The concordance rate for type 1 diabetes is about 25-50%. There may be an additional deficit in insulin secretion in type 2, which can worsen over time and eventually require insulin treatment. Certain ethnicities (African Americans, Hispanic/Latino Americans, Native Americans, and Asian Americans) have a higher predisposition to develop type 2 diabetes.

Maturity Onset Diabetes of the Young (MODY) is a monogenic autosomal dominant form of diabetes (50% of the offspring are affected), with onset in late childhood or early adulthood. It affects about 5% of diabetics in the U.S. MODY has several subtypes due to different genetic mutations, but all appear to involve an impairment of insulin secretion.

It is estimated that about 11% of the U.S. population has diabetes, about 90-95% of which have type 2. Diabetes can lead to many medical problems (**Fig. 2-4**).

Figure 2-5 lists the symptoms and signs in common or differing in type 1 and type 2 diabetes.

Diagnosis of Diabetes

Diabetes is diagnosed through a combination of clinical signs and medical tests:

- Family history of diabetes
- Clinical signs and symptoms (**Fig. 2-5**)
- **Fasting Plasma Glucose.** Glucose ≥ 126 mg/dL after an overnight fast on two separate occasions suggests diabetes. (Prediabetes: blood glucose 100-125 mg/dL)
- **Random Plasma Glucose** ≥ 200 mg/dL with typical symptoms of diabetes
- **Oral Glucose Tolerance Test**. Blood glucose is measured before and two hours after consuming a sugary solution. Glucose ≥ 200 mg/dL suggests diabetes. (Prediabetes: 140-199 mg/dL)
- **Glycated Hemoglobin (HbA1c)**. Excess glucose normally enters red blood cells and links up (glycates) with hemoglobin. This glycated hemoglobin (HbA1c) is relatively slow to build up and slow to disappear and can be measured as an index of average blood glucose over the past 2-3 months. An HbA1c level ≥ 6.5% suggest diabetes. (Prediabetes: 5.7%-6.4%)
- The presence of **pancreatic autoantibodies** supports the diagnosis of type 1.
- **C-peptide** levels (a measure of insulin production) are low or undetectable in type 1 diabetes, where insulin is not produced. C-peptide is also low in the hypoglycemia of insulin overdose, as opposed to hypoglycemia from increased insulin secretion, where insulin is synthesized in the body.

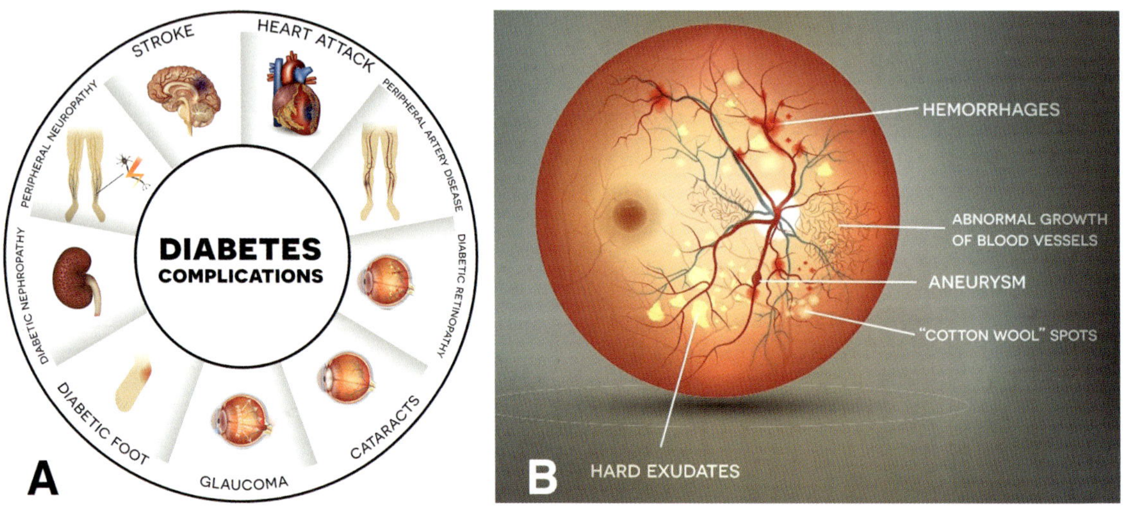

Fig. 2-4. A. Diabetes complications. B. Diabetic retinopathy.

FIGURE 2-5. SYMPTOMS AND SIGNS OF TYPE 1 AND TYPE 2 DIABETES

Common to Both Type 1 and Type 2 Diabetes:

- Hyperglycemia
- Frequent urination (**polyuria**), dehydration, and thirst (**polydipsia**). (The body attempts to remove excess glucose from the blood, leading to increased urine production, loss of body water, and thirst.)
- Increased hunger (**polyphagia**). (The body cannot utilize glucose effectively, leading to hunger.)
- Fatigue and weakness. (Cells can't get enough glucose for energy.)
- Dry mouth (dehydration)
- Blurred vision. (High sugar can pull fluid from the lens.)
- Foot ulcers (slow-healing wounds or frequent infections. Diabetes can impair immune cell function and reduce blood flow by damaging blood vessels and nerves. Also, decreased sensation in the feet from peripheral neuropathy can make it difficult for individuals to detect injuries.)

Long-term Complications:

- Glaucoma and cataracts
- Diabetic retinopathy
- Peripheral artery disease. (The impact on circulation reduces blood flow to the extremities.)
- Heart attack and stroke
- Peripheral neuropathy (perhaps from decreased blood flow to the nerves or chronic inflammation)
- Diabetic nephropathy

More Common in Type 1:

- Rapid onset (symptoms may arise in a few weeks or months; autoimmune-related)
- Diabetic Ketoacidosis (DKA). (In the absence of glucose utilization, the body breaks down fat to ketones for energy. In type 2, insulin levels are usually high enough to prevent excess accumulation of ketones.)
- Hyperkalemia. (Insulin normally drives potassium into cells, with hyperkalemia in the absence of insulin. Also, ketones are acidic and potassium leaves cells in exchange for H+ ions.)
- Nausea, vomiting, and abdominal pain (may have to do with coinciding autoimmune neuropathy that causes gastroparesis (delayed stomach emptying) in type 1 as well as the absence of insulin, which plays a role in regulating GI motility; insulin resistance in type 2 diabetes can also hinder motility of the gastrointestinal tract.)
- Fruity-smelling breath (ketones in ketoacidosis)
- Rapid breathing (an attempt by the body to reduce the acidosis from ketones in ketoacidosis)
- Weight loss more common than weight gain. (The body breaks down fat and muscle tissue for energy in the absence of insulin.)
- Younger age (due to its autoimmune nature and genetic factors)

More Common in Type 2:

- Gradual onset. (Symptoms may not be noticeable for years.)
- Insulin resistance. (Despite adequate or high insulin, the body doesn't respond to it.)
- Obesity or weight gain more common than weight loss. Over 75% of type 2 diabetics are obese. (Obesity occurs partly because the increased insulin in type 2 diabetes can still promote fat storage and inhibit fat breakdown.)
- Older age. (Type 2 is more common in middle-aged and older individuals.)
- *Acanthosis nigricans* (dark, thick, velvety patches of skin typically in skin folds, believed related to high insulin levels in insulin resistance)

Treatment of Diabetes

General measures in managing diabetes include:

- Blood glucose monitoring by fingerstick tests or glucose monitoring systems
- Carbohydrate counting and meal planning. Portion control.
- The **glycemic index** is a ranking system that measures how quickly carbohydrates in food raise blood sugar levels compared to a reference food, e.g., pure glucose or white bread. Complex carbohydrates that are high in fiber have a lower glycemic index. These include whole grains (e.g., whole wheat bread, brown rice, and oats), legumes, fruits, and vegetables. These carbohydrates are digested more slowly, resulting in a slower and more controlled rise in blood sugar levels. Foods with a high glycemic index

cause a more rapid and significant increase in blood sugar levels. Balanced meals that include carbohydrates, protein, and healthy fats slow down the absorption of glucose.

- Reduced added sugars
- Regular meal timing to regulate blood sugar levels
- Regular physical activity
- Education and self-management – e.g., learning how to monitor blood sugar levels and administer insulin
- Regular medical checkups (including blood pressure, cholesterol, kidney function, and eye and foot health)
- Addressing potential complications that may arise from chronic high blood sugar
- Hemoglobin A1c test, usually measured every 3-6 months, provides a monitor of the effectiveness of glucose control and risk for diabetic complications, such as retinopathy, nephropathy, neuropathy, and cardiovascular disease.
- For prediabetes, preventive measures are recommended: healthy diet, increased physical activity, and maintaining a healthy weight, with regular monitoring and follow-up with a healthcare professional.
- **Medication for type 1 diabetes** consists of lifetime insulin replacement through daily injections (syringes or pens) or an insulin pump (**Fig. 2-6**):

Rapid-acting and ***short-acting insulins*** begin to work within about 15-30 minutes after injection and peak within about 1-4 hours, lasting about 3-8 hrs. Generally, they are taken just before or right after meals to control post-meal sugar spikes or to correct high blood sugars that are not in the target range between meals. These include *insulin lispro* (*Humalog*), *insulin aspart* (*Novolog* or *NovoRapid*), *insulin glulisine* (*Apidra*), *regular insulin* (chemically identical to natural human insulin), *Humulin*, and *Novolin*.

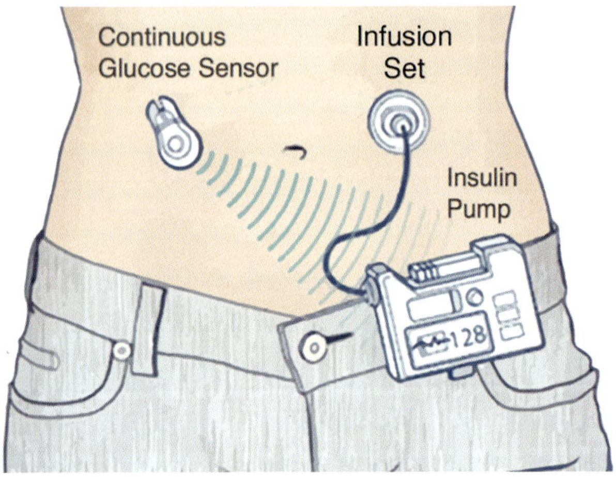

Fig. 2-6. One type of insulin pump. A continuous glucose sensor tracks glucose levels through the day and night and sends wireless signals to an insulin pump receiver, which uses an algorithm to determine the appropriate insulin delivery rate. Insulin is pumped to the infusion set, which delivers the insulin subcutaneously via a fine needle or canula.

Intermediate-acting insulin helps cover the periods between meals. It usually starts working within 1-2 hours, peaks in 4-6 hrs and can last up to 12-18 hrs. It is used to provide background insulin coverage throughout the day (e.g., *NPH, Lente*).

Long-acting insulin provides a continuing basal insulin level throughout the day and night (**Fig. 2-7**). It typically starts working within 1-2 hours, has no pronounced peak, and can last for approximately 24 hours or longer, e.g., *insulin glargine (Lantus, Basaglar, Toujeo)*, and *insulin detemir*. The aim is to keep glucose levels steady, without hyperglycemia or hypoglycemia.

Ultra-Long-Acting Insulin can last up to 36-48 hours, e.g., *insulin degludec (Tresiba).*

Current interest focuses on insulin forms requiring only once-weekly injection (e.g., insulin *icodec*), for type 1 and type 2 diabetes. This offers the important convenience of having to make only 52 injections/year rather than 365.

These medications can be given in different combinations depending on the individual's needs.

Islet cell autotransplantation to the liver of islet cells removed during a pancreatectomy (e.g., for chronic pancreatitis) can allow insulin independence. This procedure is not typically done for type 1 or type 2 diabetes due to the autoimmune process that kills the patient's beta pancreatic cells in type 1, and the resistance to insulin in type 2. However, cells from a donor pancreas, combined with immunosuppression

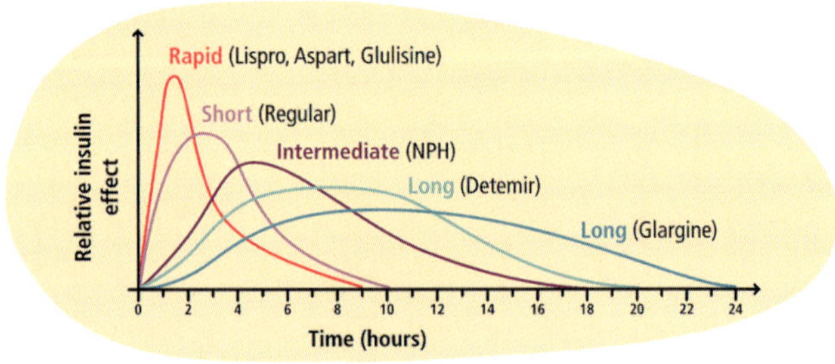

Fig. 2-7. Timing of action of the insulin types.

is a possibility under investigation for type 1 diabetes. Pancreatic transplant is sometimes used in conjunction with kidney transplantation in patients who have both type 1 diabetes and kidney failure.

- **Type 2 diabetic medications** (**Fig. 2-8**) are mainly oral:

  Metformin reduces glucose production in the liver by inhibiting the enzyme glucose-6-phosphatase, which is important in releasing glucose into the bloodstream; it also increases insulin sensitivity in peripheral tissues, improving the uptake and use of glucose by peripheral tissues, such as muscle and fat cells. Metformin does not cause hypoglycemia. However, it can increase the risk of lactic acidosis and is generally contraindicated or used with great caution in conditions that predispose to lactic acidosis, such as severe renal or liver disease.

  Sulfonoureas (e.g., *glimepiride, glipizide, glyburide*) stimulate insulin release from the pancreas and increase insulin sensitivity in peripheral tissues.

  Meglitinides (glinides) (e.g., *repaglinide, nateglinide*) stimulate insulin release from the pancreas, particularly when blood glucose levels are high.

  Thiazoliginediones (TZDs, glitazones) (e.g., *pioglitazone, rosiglitazone*) increase insulin sensitivity in the body cells, improving the uptake and utilization of glucose. They also reduce hepatic glucose production and can increase blood levels of HDL (good) cholesterol and decrease levels of triglycerides.

  Glucagon-like peptide-1 (GLP-1) receptor agonists ("incretin mimetics")(e.g., *exenatide, liraglutide, dulaglutide, lixisenatide, semaglutide [Ozempic]*) mimic the effects of intestinal GLP-1. Some (*albiglutide, dulaglutide, exenatide long-acting release*) last as long as a week. *Trizepatide* is a combined GIP/GLP-1 receptor agonist. Both GIP (Glucose-Dependent Insulinotropic Peptide) and GLP-1 are *incretins*, which stimulate insulin production and release from the pancreas when blood glucose levels are high, suppress glucagon secretion, and slow gastric emptying, delaying the absorption of glucose. They also promote a feeling of fullness and enable weight loss. In some people, GLP-1 receptor agonists are used for weight loss. These medications are generally given by injection, although semaglutide has an oral formulation.

  Dipeptidyl peptidase-4 (DPP-4) inhibitors (gliptins) (e.g., *sitagliptin, saxagliptin, linagliptin*) inhibit the enzymatic activity of DPP-4, an enzyme that degrades intestinal incretin hormones, e.g., glucagon-like peptide-1 (GLP-1) and glucose-dependent insulinotropic polypeptide (GIP). The drug inhibition of DPP-4 increases the levels of GLP-1 and GIP.

  Sodium-glucose cotransporter-2 (SGLT2) inhibitors (e.g., *canagliflozin, dapagliflozin, empagliflozin, ertugliflozin, ipragliflozin*) prevent the kidneys from reabsorbing glucose, thereby increasing excretion of glucose in the urine. This also has a mild diuretic effect that can help people with heart failure by reducing fluid retention.

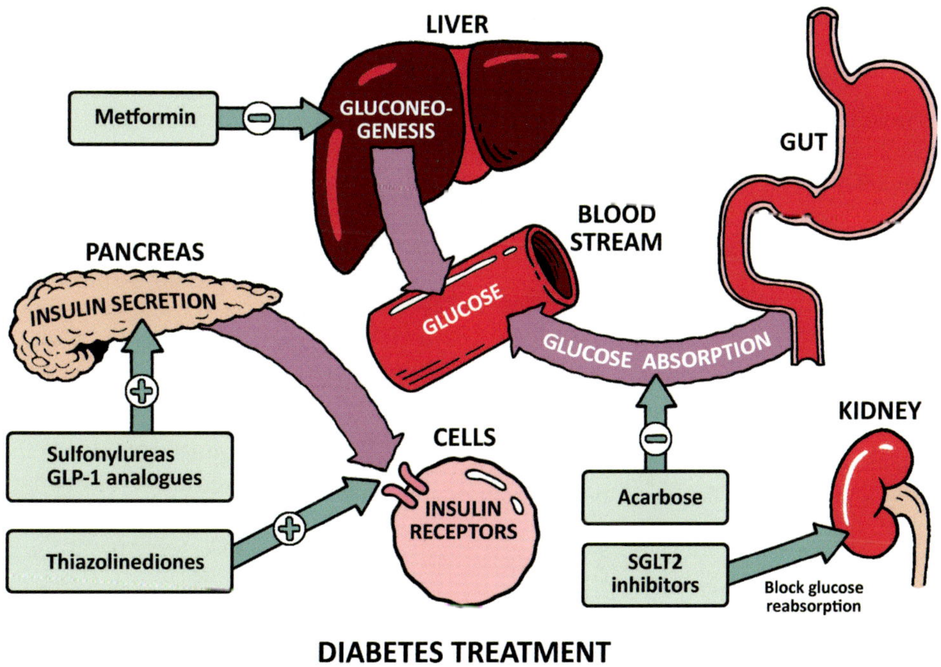

Fig. 2-8 Diabetes treatment.

FIGURE 2-9. CAUSES OF HYPERGLYCEMIA

- Diabetes type 1 or type 2
- Pancreatic disease or surgery (e.g., chronic pancreatitis, pancreatic cancer, pancreatic surgery)
- High carbohydrate intake
- Lack of physical activity
- Medications. Some interfere with insulin release (e.g., thiazides, phenytoin, cyclosporine) while others cause insulin resistance (e.g., glucocorticoids, oral contraceptive pills).
- Hormonal imbalances. Excess glucagon, cortisol, growth hormone, epinephrine, thyroid hormone, estrogen or progesterone also cause elevated blood glucose, by either increasing peripheral resistance to insulin or impairing insulin release from the beta cells.
- Chronic alcoholic pancreatitis (causes loss of beta cells)
- *Gestational diabetes* may have to do with hormonal changes; it usually disappears after childbirth, but type 2 diabetes is more likely to develop later, within 5-10 years.

Alpha-glucosidase inhibitors (e.g., *acarbose*) slow down the action of enzymes in the small intestine that break down glucose, resulting in a slower rise in blood glucose after meals.

Insulin (injection) may be added in type 2 diabetes in cases where blood sugar is not well-managed with oral medication. While insulin levels may be elevated in the early stages of type 2 diabetes as a response to insulin resistance, eventually as type 2 progresses, the beta cells in the pancreas may become exhausted keeping up with the increased demand for insulin. This can lead to a decline in insulin levels in the blood, which may be approached by adding insulin to the regimen.

Not every instance of hyperglycemia has to do with type 1 or type 2 diabetes. There are other causes, described in **Figure 2-9**.

Diabetic Ketoacidosis (DKA)

DKA is characterized by the accumulation of ketones in the blood, typically in individuals with uncontrolled type 1 diabetes (although it can occur in type 2), when blood sugar levels are very high (usually >250 mg/dL) and there is a lack of insulin, sometimes from missed insulin doses or insulin pump failure. Infection and excess alcohol, as well as physical or emotional stress can trigger it.

The high sugar can cause dehydration, electrolyte imbalances, confusion and even coma. The dehydration occurs partly because there is too much excess glucose in the urine to be adequately reabsorbed. This has an osmotic effect that pulls in water, which is excreted.

Acidosis caused by the acidotic ketones (**Fig. 2-3B**) can disrupt normal cellular functions and adversely affect organ systems. The breathing may be heavy (*Kussmaul breathing*) to clear CO_2 and reduce the acidosis. Acidosis, as measured by arterial blood gases, can also cause high blood potassium (hyperkalemia) due to potassium leaving cells in exchange for H+ ions. (Hyperkalemia may also be due to lack of insulin, which normally drives potassium into cells.) Initially, there may be a hypokalemia from potassium loss in the kidney due to osmotic diuresis in the kidney tubules, with reduced potassium reabsorption, but as the acidosis worsens, the blood becomes hyperkalemic from exchange of H+ for potassium in body cells.

At the start of treatment for DKA, potassium in the blood may at first be high (hyperkalemia) as potassium in the cells exchanges with H+ ions in the acidotic blood. But potassium may then fall (hypokalemia) as a result of the insulin treatment, which drives potassium into the cells.

Excess insulin therapy for DKA can cause hypoglycemia, with cerebral edema, confusion and coma from rapid osmotic changes. Hypokalemia may cause abnormal heart rhythms and cardiovascular collapse. Kidney function may be impaired, with decreased urine output and potential kidney damage.

Since insulin drives both glucose and potassium into cells, the blood potassium as well as blood glucose and the acidity of ketoacidosis need to be monitored carefully in DKA, with administration of bicarbonate if needed (to counteract the acidosis) and potassium when low, with continual blood test monitoring. Fluid replacement to correct dehydration, along with insulin administration, electrolyte replacement, acidosis correction, and treatment of underlying triggers, e.g., infections and illness, are important parts of the treatment of DKA.

Hyperosmolar Nonketotic Coma (HNC)

Hyperosmolar nonketotic coma (HNC) is a complication of type 2 diabetes marked by very high levels of glucose, often > 600 mg/dL, even more than in DKA. Like DKA, HNC incurs hyperglycemia, dehydration and altered mental status. HNC, though differs from DKA in several ways:

- There is no significant ketosis in HNC, since type 2 diabetes is a disease of insulin resistance rather than insulin lack. There is generally enough insulin in HNC to prevent the breakdown of fat into ketones.
- Acidosis and fruity breath are not prominent in HNC, since there is no excess of ketones, which are acidic and smell fruity.

- HNC is not marked by the deep Kussmaul breathing of DKA, which is needed to help correct the acidosis.

The general treatment approach in HNC resembles that in DKA, except:

- The dehydration is usually worse in HNC and may need a more aggressive approach to rehydrate.
- Insulin needs may differ in the two conditions, and HNC may need a less aggressive initial approach to insulin therapy.
- Ketone monitoring and correction of acidosis are generally not a focus in treating HNC due to the lack of ketones.

Hypoglycemia

Figure 2-10 reviews the symptoms, signs, and potential causes of hypoglycemia.

Treatment of Hypoglycemia

- Consume fast-acting carbohydrates (glucose tablets or gel; fruit juice, regular soda; hard candies or glucose sweets).
- Repeat blood after 15 minutes to recheck blood sugar levels.
- Eat a balanced meal or snack once blood glucose levels have returned to normal.
- Inject glucagon when the patient can't consume oral carbohydrates or is unconscious.
- Use intravenous glucose if available. Draw a blood sample for glucose before glucose administration to confirm that the problem just treated was actually hypoglycemia.

Glucagon

Glucagon, produced by pancreatic alpha cells, acts opposite to insulin. Glucagon promotes glucose

FIGURE 2-10. HYPOGLYCEMIA
Symptoms and Signs of Hypoglycemia
• Shaking and trembling. (The release of stress hormones like epinephrine and norepinephrine in response to low blood sugar helps raise blood glucose levels but also generates a sympathetic nervous system response.)
• Sweating (sympathetic nervous system response)
• Dizziness and lightheadedness. (The brain isn't getting enough glucose; also, there is the sympathetic nervous system response.)
• Confusion and difficulty concentrating. (The brain isn't getting enough glucose.)
• Hunger. (The brain interprets low sugar as an energy deficit and signals the body to increase food intake.)
• Weakness, fatigue (low glucose = less available energy)
• Headache. (Epinephrine can cause blood vessel constriction, followed by dilation to increase blood flow to the brain, leading to headache.)
• Blurred vision. (Hypoglycemia can cause osmotic changes in lens shape.)
• Mood changes. (Proper brain function depends on adequate glucose.)
• Rapid heartbeat (sympathetic response)
Causes of Hypoglycemia
• Diabetes medications may lower blood glucose levels excessively (the usual cause).
• Insulinoma
• Excess physical activity
• Sepsis can cause hypoglycemia, partly due to increased metabolic rate that can deplete glucose stores.
• Skipping meals
• Excess alcohol consumption. (Alcohol interferes with the liver's ability to produce glucose.)
• Deficiencies in hormones that normally raise blood glucose (e.g., glucagon, epinephrine, cortisol, or growth hormone)
• Liver diseases (through decreased ability to store glycogen, produce glucose, or clear insulin)
• Kidney disorders (through reduced gluconeogenesis, insulin clearance and glucose reabsorption)
• Metabolic disorders: Including glycogen storage diseases (decreased ability to store or break down glycogen to glucose); disorders of fatty acid oxidation (the body can't break down fatty acids to glucose); genetic disorders of gluconeogenesis.
• Postprandial hypoglycemia. (Some people get hypoglycemic a few hours after eating a high-carbohydrate meal, which may involve an exaggerated insulin response to the meal.)
• Autoimmune hypoglycemia with inappropriate activation of insulin receptors

release from the liver through glycogen breakdown (*glycogenolysis*), and glucose production from non-carbohydrate sources — glycerol and amino acids (*gluconeogenesis*). Glucagon also stimulates lipolysis, breaking down triglycerides from adipose (fat) tissue to fatty acids, to be used as an energy source other than glucose. The reciprocal relationship between insulin and glucagon helps maintain glucose balance.

Hyperglucagonemia

Glucagon can be secreted in excess, leading to symptoms of hyperglycemia. This may occur with a glucagonoma or pancreatic alpha-cell hyperplasia. Glucagonoma may be associated with a peculiar skin rash, *necrolytic migratory erythema*, and with *excess clotting*. It may also be associated with *Multiple Endocrine Neoplasia Type1 (MEN1)*, a hereditary disorder characterized by the development of tumors in multiple endocrine glands, most commonly the parathyroid glands, pancreatic islet cells, and anterior pituitary gland.

Blood tests can measure glucagon as well as insulin and other hormones to rule out MEN1. Imaging studies (e.g., CT scan, MRI, or ultrasound) can visualize the pancreas and identify tumors or pancreatic hyperplasia. Genetic testing can detect mutations in the GCG gene, which encodes for glucagon.

Treatment of hyperglucagonemia is aimed at addressing the underlying cause (e.g., surgery to remove a glucagonoma), symptom management (e.g., reducing hyperglycemia, or palliating skin problems with creams or ointments), and diet regulation for optimal glucose control.

Hypoglucagonemia

Hypoglucagonemia can result from pancreatic alpha-cell deficiency, pancreatitis, and pancreatic surgery. The symptoms include hypoglycemia, as well as problems in growth and development when the hypoglycemia is chronic since childhood. The measurement of glucagon levels, as well as genetic testing for the GCG gene may be diagnostic. The treatment involves addressing the cause (pancreatic disorders, genetic mutations, autoimmune conditions), as well as glucagon replacement therapy (injection or nasal spray).

Somatostatin

Somatostatin is mainly produced in the pancreas, hypothalamus, stomach and small intestine. It has diverse inhibitory effects. Somatostatin inhibits the secretion of growth hormone, insulin, glucagon, thyroid-stimulating hormone, and various gastrointestinal hormones, including gastrin and secretin. In doing so, somatostatin helps prevent excessive hormone production. Also, somatostatin:

- Slows down stomach and intestinal motility. This allows more time for the thorough digestion and absorption of nutrients. Somatostatin also reduces the rate of secretion of digestive enzymes and inhibits the release of bile from the gallbladder, helping to match the digestive capacity to the reduced motility in the intestines.
- Modulates blood flow by vasoconstriction, reducing blood flow to non-essential areas and prioritizing blood flow to essential organs, like the brain and heart.
- Acts as a neurotransmitter in the nervous system, helping to regulate neuronal activity and neurotransmission. It is involved in inhibitory signaling, counteracting the effects of excitatory neurotransmitters to maintain balanced neuronal activity. This includes modulating pain signals and acting as an analgesic. In the pituitary gland, somatostatin inhibits the secretion of growth hormone, thyroid-stimulating hormone, and ACTH.
- Affects immune function. It can dampen excessive immune activation and reduce inflammation.

Excess somatostatin secretion (**somatostatinoma syndrome**) causes symptoms of diabetes from impaired insulin secretion. It may also cause gallstones, malabsorption, weight loss, abdominal pain, nausea, vomiting, and chronic diarrhea from its effect on the GI tract. The excess somatostatin may result from a somatostatinoma of the pancreas or other parts of the GI tract, or from a neuroendocrine tumor.

The **diagnosis** of somatostatinoma includes:

- Blood tests for levels of somatostatin, or insulin, glucagon, and gastrin (which may be decreased from excess somatostatin)
- Imaging studies, including CT scan, MRI, or *somatostatin receptor scintigraphy:* A radioactive somatostatin analogue (e.g., *octreotide*) binds to somatostatin receptors on somatostatinoma tumor cells and can be detected by a special gamma camera.
- Biopsy to confirm somatostatinoma or other tumor types that secrete excess somatostatin

The **treatment** of a somatostatinoma may involve surgery or chemotherapy, as well as supportive care for the symptoms.

Somatostatin deficiency, a rare condition, may result from removal of somatostatin-secreting tissue (e.g., pancreatic surgery, pancreatic tumors, genetic disorders), radiation or chemotherapy, autoimmune disorders that target somatostatin-producing cells, and pancreatitis. It can lead to the overproduction of hormones normally inhibited by somatostatin, such as growth hormone, insulin, glucagon, and various gastrointestinal hormones.

The **diagnosis** of somatostatin deficiency can be narrowed by assessing the levels of hormones regulated by somatostatin (such as insulin and growth hormone), imaging studies of the pancreas or hypothalamus for any abnormalities that could cause somatostatin deficiency, and genetic testing. It is important to rule out other possible causes of the patient's symptoms, like pancreatic disorders, GI diseases, or malabsorption syndromes that may present with similar features.

Treatment of somatostatin deficiency may involve:

- Management of the symptoms
- Somatostatin analogues (e.g., *octreotide, lanreotide*), which can mimic the inhibitory effects of somatostatin on hormone secretion, thereby reducing the excess secretion of other hormones.
- Follow-up with periodic blood tests, imaging studies or other assessments

The pancreatic and other hormones work together to regulate blood glucose levels and ensure that the body has enough energy to meet its demands, especially during stress, physical activity, or fasting. An imbalance in these hormonal responses can lead to diabetes or other metabolic disorders.

Pancreatic Polypeptide

Pancreatic polypeptide is secreted by PP cells in the islets of Langerhans. It inhibits the secretion of *exocrine* enzymes in the pancreas and reduces the rate of gastric emptying and intestinal motility, creating a feeling of fullness after eating. PP can also inhibit *endocrine* cell secretion in the pancreas, suppressing the release of insulin, glucagon, and somatostatin. Presently, PP is used more as a diagnostic tool to assess pancreatic function than as a therapeutic agent. Reduced PP levels may suggest impaired pancreatic function. There are also rare pancreatic PP tumors (PPomas, glucagonomas), where measurement of PP levels can help in their diagnosis and monitoring.

Which Hormones Increase Blood Glucose?

- **Glucagon**, produced by the pancreatic alpha cells
- **Cortisol**, produced by the adrenal cortex
- **Epinephrine (Adrenaline)/Norepinephrine (Noradrenaline)**, produced by the adrenal medulla
- **Growth hormone (Somatotropin)**, produced by the pituitary gland
- **Thyroid hormones** (T3 and T4), produced by the thyroid gland
- **Somatostatin**, produced by the Delta cells of the pancreas. (Its inhibitory effect on insulin secretion tends to be stronger than its inhibitory effect on glucagon secretion, with a tendency toward increasing blood glucose.)

Which Hormones Decrease Blood Glucose?

- **Insulin**, secreted by the beta cells of the pancreas
- **Amylin**. Amylin is co-secreted with insulin by the beta cells of the pancreas. It slows the rate at which the liver releases glucose into the bloodstream after eating, thereby reducing post-meal spikes in blood glucose levels.
- **Incretins (GLP-1 and GIP)**. Glucagon-like peptide 1 (GLP-1) and gastric inhibitory peptide (GIP) are hormones released from the intestines in response to food intake. They stimulate insulin secretion when blood glucose levels are high.
- **Somatostatin** in some contexts can lower blood glucose by inhibiting the release of growth hormone and glucagon.

Chapter 3 **Thyroid Gland**

The thyroid gland (**Fig. 3-1**) is a small, butterfly-shaped gland in the front of the neck, just below the Adam's apple. It produces two kinds of hormones:

- Thyroid hormone (T4 and T3)
- Calcitonin

Thyroid Hormone

Thyroid hormone consists of thyroxine (T4) and triiodothyronine (T3), which act on almost every body tissue and have multiple functions:

- Metabolism Regulation: They increase the body's metabolic rate; the cells use energy more quickly.
- Heart Function: They increase heart rate and cardiac contractility.
- Development and Growth: They are important for normal growth and development in children.
- Thermogenesis: They help regulate body temperature by generating heat.
- Nervous System: They increase alertness and reflexes by enhancing the effects of neurotransmitters like epinephrine and norepinephrine.
- Respiratory Function: They stimulate breathing (since more oxygen is needed).
- Bone Health: They assist in bone development and in maintaining bone density.
- Cholesterol and Lipid Metabolism: They help maintain healthy levels of cholesterol and other lipids.
- Gastrointestinal Function: They increase the rate of digestion by stimulating the muscles of the GI tract.
- Muscle Function: They increase muscle strength and rate of contraction and aid in muscle development, maintenance and repair.
- Red Blood Cell Production: They stimulate the production of red blood cells, enhancing oxygen transport.
- Skin Health: They help maintain healthy skin.

Thyroxine (T4) is the main hormone secreted by the thyroid gland. It is converted in the peripheral tissues to **triiodothyronine (T3)**, the more active form of thyroid hormone. Both T3 and T4 help regulate body metabolism by converting food into energy. The energy is used for growth and development, heat production, and the functioning of various organs, including the heart, brain, liver, muscles, bone, reproductive organs, and digestive system, which depend on precise amounts of T3 and T4 in the bloodstream.

The thyroid gland is regulated by the hypothalamus and the pituitary gland. The hypothalamus produces **thyrotropin-releasing hormone (TRH)**, which signals the pituitary gland to release **thyroid-stimulating hormone (TSH).** TSH then stimulates the thyroid gland to produce and release T3 and T4 hormones into the bloodstream (**Fig 3-1**).

Excess amounts of T3 and T4 in the blood feed back to suppress the hypothalamus' secretion of TRH and the pituitary gland's release of TSH (**Fig. 3-1**).

THYROID HORMONES

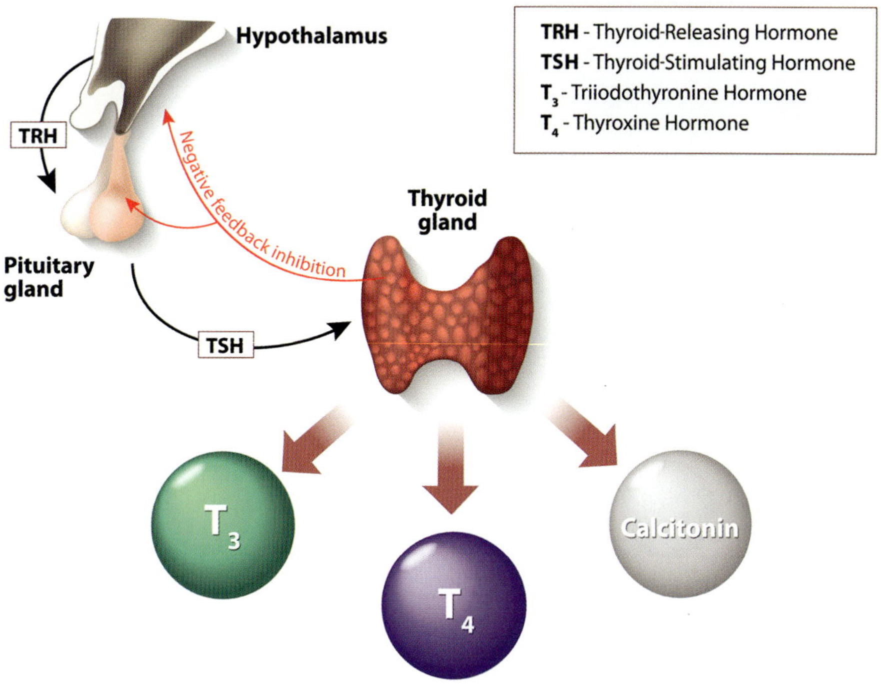

Fig. 3-1. Thyroid hormones and their feedback to the hypothalamus and pituitary gland.

Too little T3 and T4 causes the pituitary to secrete more TSH. This type of feedback mechanism is common throughout the endocrine system. It is vital to maintain T3 and T4 at optimal blood levels. Disease manifests when the levels of thyroid hormone are either too high (**hyperthyroidism**) or too low (**hypothyroidism**).

Hyperthyroidism

In **primary hyperthyroidism**, the problem is an intrinsically overactive thyroid gland. T3 and T4 levels are high, but TSH levels are low, due to negative feedback of T3 and T4 on the hypothalamus and pituitary gland, which then lower the production of TSH (**Fig. 3-2**).

In **secondary hyperthyroidism**, the problem lies with the pituitary gland, which oversecretes TSH. As a result, the T3 and T4 are high, but so is the TSH, which the pituitary independently oversecretes.

In **tertiary hyperthyroidism**, the problem lies with the hypothalamus, which secretes too much thyroid-releasing hormone (TRH), which in turn stimulates the pituitary to produce too much TSH, and hence results in hyperthyroidism.

Synthesis of Thyroid Hormone

Within the thyroid gland, **thyroglobulin** serves as a storage protein for T4 and T3 within the viscous colloid of thyroid follicles, which are lined by a single layer of secreting follicular ("cuboidal") cells. Once outside the thyroid, in the bloodstream, T4 and T3 bind to **thyroxine-binding globulin (TBG)(Fig. 3-3)** for transport. *Free* T3, which is not bound to thyroxine-binding globulin, is the active portion of thyroid hormone and the most reliable for measurement of active thyroid hormone in blood tests. The measurement of *Total* T3, which includes thyroxine-binding globulin is not as useful, since TBG levels can be influenced by various factors, such as hormonal changes, liver function, and certain medications.

In peripheral tissues, T4 is converted to T3 by the removal of an iodine atom. T3 enters target cells more readily than T4. Once inside the cell, T3 binds to thyroid hormone receptors in the nucleus. (Steroid hormones also tend to act in the cell nucleus, as opposed to protein receptors at the cell membrane, the way used by other hormones.) These nuclear receptors regulate gene expression. The result is an increase in metabolic rate

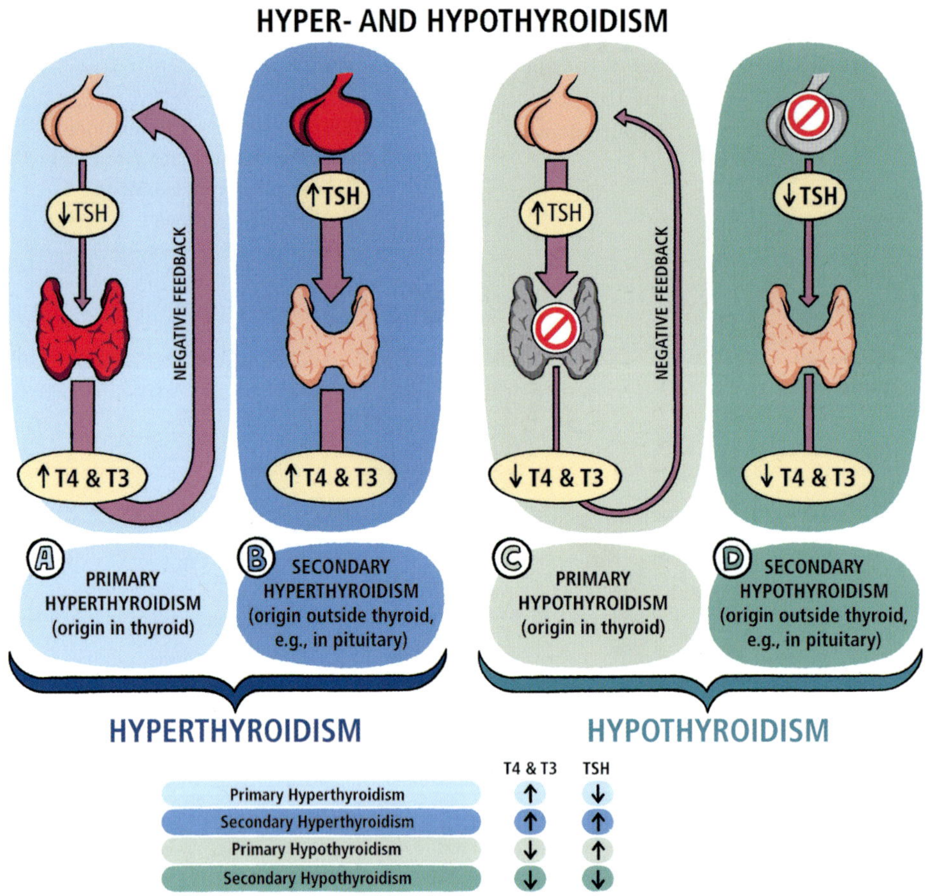

Fig. 3-2. Thyroid-Stimulating Hormone levels in hyperthyroidism and hypothyroidism. (Modified from Berkowitz, A. Clinical Pathophysiology Made Ridiculously Simple. Medmaster.)

and oxygen consumption, enhanced energy production, and stimulation of the breakdown of fats (lipolysis) and carbohydrates (glycolysis). Thyroid hormones also promote protein synthesis and growth, affect cardiovascular function, and influence the development and function of various tissues and organs.

Both hyperthyroidism and hypothyroidism are more common in women. The signs and symptoms of hyperthyroidism largely relate to an increase in metabolism from the increased secretion of thyroid hormone:

- Weight loss even with increased appetite
- Rapid heartbeat and palpitations
- Heat intolerance and sweating (excess heat from increased metabolism)
- Nervousness and anxiety
- Fatigue and muscle weakness (the body can't keep up with metabolic demands)
- Tremors and muscle hyperactivity (influence of thyroid hormone on the central nervous system)
- Frequent bowel movements
- Menstrual irregularities (effect on sex hormone production and availability)
- Insomnia (nervous system effect)
- Exophthalmos (*proptosis*). There is bulging of the eyes with exposure of the white of the sclera above the cornea, giving the eyes the appearance of a stare (**Fig. 3-4A**). There may be double vision (*diplopia*). This is seen mainly in **Graves' disease**, an autoimmune condition and the most common cause of hyperthyroidism.
- Enlarged thyroid (*goiter*) (**Fig. 3-4B**)
- *Lid retraction*. The upper lid appears retracted. This may be due to the combination of proptosis of the eye and sympathetic overactivity of the upper lid.
- *Lid lag*. The upper eyelid lags in following the eye on downward gaze (may result from sympathetic hyperactivity that makes the ocular muscles move more rapidly than the upper eyelid on downward gaze, or to sympathetic overactivity of the upper lid).

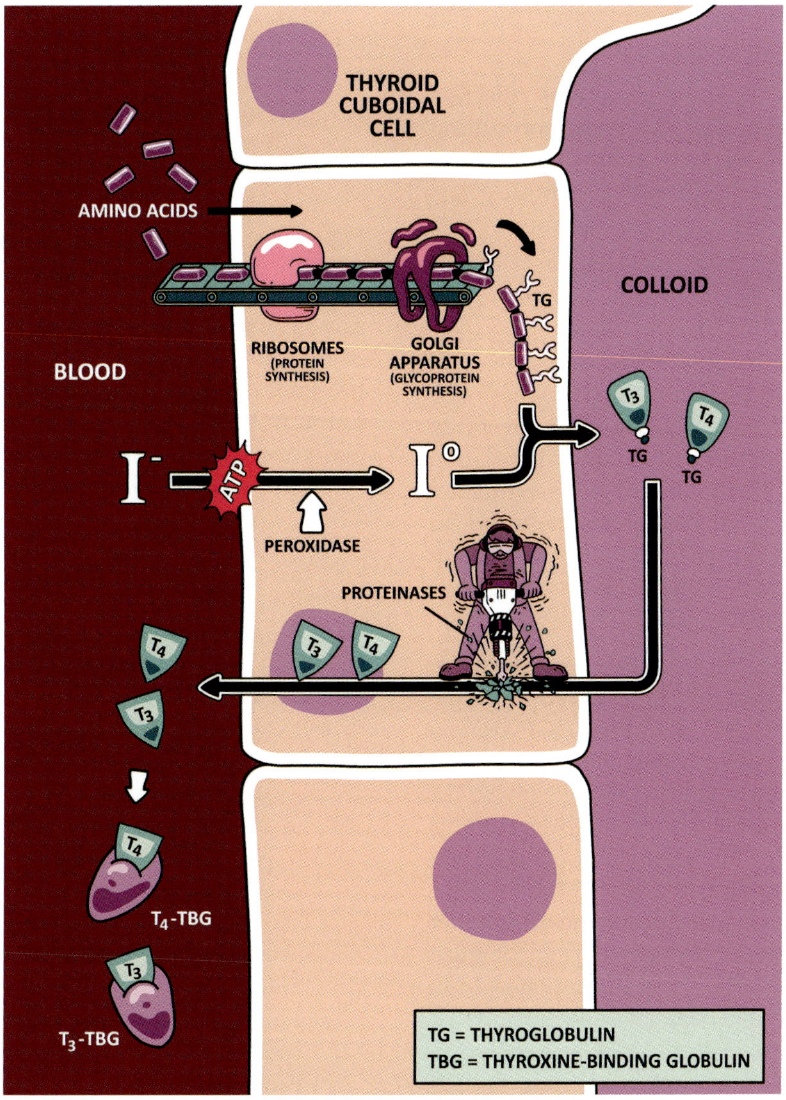

Fig. 3-3. Synthesis of thyroid hormone in the thyroid cuboidal (follicular) cell. (From Goldberg, S. Clinical Physiology Made Ridiculously Simple. Medmaster.)

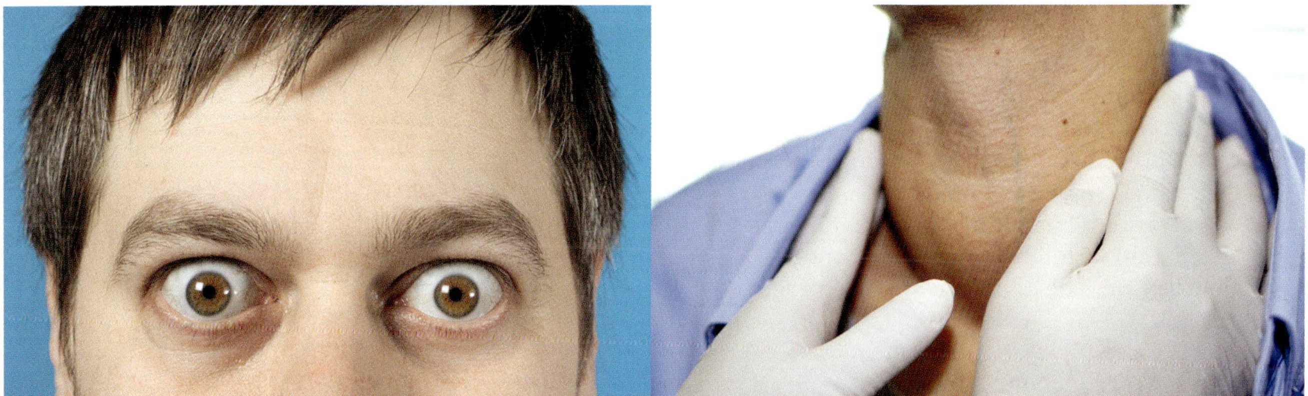

Fig. 3-4. Graves' disease. A. Exophthalmos. B. Goiter.

In addition, there may be several other peculiar manifestations of hyperthyroidism:

- *Pretibial myxedema* (mainly in Graves' disease, where an autoimmune reaction causes non-pitting edema in the lower legs, with accumulation of *hyaluronic acid*, particularly over the tibia)
- *Osteoporosis.* (Excess thyroid hormone can accelerate bone turnover.)

Causes of Hyperthyroidism

- *Graves' disease*, an autoimmune condition, is the most common cause of hyperthyroidism. It is mediated by **thyroid-stimulating immunoglobulin** (TSI), which mimics the action of thyroid-stimulating hormone (TSH). Constant thyroid stimulation and overproduction of thyroid hormones can lead to the enlargement of the thyroid. The patient often has a diffuse, nontender goiter, as well as exophthalmos (**Fig. 3-4**).

Regarding the exophthalmos (Graves' Eye Disease; Thyroid Eye Disease; TED), it is believed that the **insulin-like growth factor-1 receptors** (**IGF-1R**) on fibroblasts behind the eye are activated by **IGF-1 receptor antibodies**. (IGF-1 receptor antibodies differ from the TSI antibodies responsible for the overactive thyroid.) This induces the fibroblasts to produce hyaluronic acid and differentiate into fat, fibroblast, and myofibroblast cells, which deposit behind the eye, including the extraocular muscles and connective tissue, causing the eye to bulge. It is unclear why sometimes the process is unilateral, but it is possible that it is actually bilateral, only asymmetric and much more pronounced in one eye.

- *Toxic adenoma*. These tumors are generally benign but secrete thyroid hormone. They show up as "hot" nodules on radioactive iodine scans, rather than the diffuse lighting up of the thyroid found in Graves' disease.
- *Toxic multinodular goiter*. Abnormal nodules in the thyroid, particularly in older patients, become overactive and secrete thyroid hormone independent of TSH control. It is more common in regions where iodine deficiency is prevalent. They show up as hot nodules on thyroid scan. The goiter is typically nontender.
- *Thyroiditis*. Inflammation of the thyroid can lead to release of stored thyroid hormones into the bloodstream. The thyroid gland may be tender or nontender.
- Excess iodine intake can result in more thyroid hormone production.
- TSH-secreting pituitary tumors or excess hypothalamic secretion of thyroid-releasing hormone can cause hyperthyroidism.
- Abnormally increased TSH receptor sensitivity in the thyroid gland
- *Factitious hyperthyroidism* (from ingestion of thyroid hormone for purposes of weight loss)
- High **Human Chorionic Gonadotropin** (**hCG**) (secreted by trophoblastic tumors, cross-reacts weakly with TSH receptors)

Diagnosis of Hyperthyroidism

The history and physical exam, including the finding of thyroid nodules, provide important clues as to the presence of hyperthyroidism. (A goiter, though, can be found in both hyper- and hypothyroidism, and not in everyone with these conditions.)

Useful blood tests include:

- Elevated levels of *free* T3 and *free* T4 (the active forms of thyroid hormone, which are more reliable indicators of hyperthyroidism than the *total* T3 and T4, which includes the inactive T3 and T4 that is bound to carrier proteins, i.e., thyroxine-binding globulin)
- TSH levels are usually decreased in primary hyperthyroidism. (Excess thyroid hormone causes negative feedback on the pituitary gland.) TSH is increased, though, in secondary hyperthyroidism due to excess pituitary TSH secretion.
- Thyroid antibodies, including thyroid-stimulating immunoglobulins and thyroid peroxidase antibodies, can be detected in Graves' disease.
- Radioactive Iodine Uptake (RAIU) scan. Different patterns of uptake can help differentiate various causes of hyperthyroidism. For instance, RAIU is typically elevated locally within "hot" nodules of toxic nodular goiter, but "cold" in nonfunctioning nodules. RAIU is elevated more diffusely in Graves' disease.
- Imaging (Ultrasound, CT scan, MRI) can assess the size and shape of abnormalities in the thyroid and pituitary glands.
- Fine-needle aspiration biopsy can evaluate nodules and rule out thyroid cancer.

Treatment of Hyperthyroidism

The main aim of treatment for hyperthyroidism is the reduction of thyroid hormone levels:

- Antithyroid medications (e.g., *methimazole*, *propylthiouracil*) inhibit the production of thyroid hormone. They do not, however, have a permanent effect on thyroid function.
- Radioactive iodine therapy destroys overactive thyroid tissue.

- Thyroidectomy, subtotal or total, removes actively secreting thyroid tissue.
- Supersaturated potassium iodide (SSKI) is sometimes used 1-2 weeks before thyroid surgery, based on the principle that a large influx of iodine inhibits the thyroid gland from synthesizing thyroid hormones (the *Wolff-Chaikoff effect*). This makes surgery less risky by reducing the vascularity of the thyroid gland and preventing *thyroid storm*, a severe exacerbation of hyperthyroid symptoms.
- Radiofrequency thyroid ablation is minimally invasive; heat is used to destroy overactive thyroid nodules.
- Beta blockers (e.g., *propranolol*, *atenolol*) treat the secondary symptoms of tachycardia, tremors and anxiety.
- For TSH-secreting pituitary adenomas, treatment may include surgical removal of the adenoma, radiation therapy, or medication to suppress TSH secretion (e.g., somatostatin analogs, such as *octreotide*).
- Dopamine agonists (e.g., *cabergoline* or *bromocriptine*) can occasionally be used to decrease TSH secretion in a pituitary adenoma. Dopamine not only inhibits excessive secretion of prolactin in the pituitary gland (**Fig. 1-4**) but also inhibits TSH-secreting cells.
- The exophthalmos of Graves' disease can be treated with *teprotumumab-trbw* (*Tepezza*), a monoclonal antibody against the IGF-1 receptor on orbital fibroblasts.

Hypothyroidism

As one might expect, the signs and symptoms of hypothyroidism largely relate to a decrease in metabolism from either the decreased secretion of thyroid hormone or insensitivity to the thyroid hormone that is secreted. Hypothyroidism causes:

- Fatigue and weakness (less energy production)
- Slow heart rate
- Weight gain. (Fewer calories are burned and there may be water retention, partly from decreased renal blood flow from decreased cardiac output.)
- Cold intolerance from reduced heat production
- Constipation from slowed GI transit
- Depression and mood changes. Imbalances in thyroid hormone affect the brain, neurotransmitters, and other hormones, in addition to the stress of being sick.
- Memory and cognitive problems from reduced brain metabolism
- Menstrual irregularities. (Decreased thyroid hormone can disrupt the normal balance of reproductive hormones.)
- Dry skin and hair loss from reduced sebaceous gland function
- Goiter from increased thyroid stimulation by thyroid-stimulating hormone (TSH) in an effort to boost lagging hormone production in primary hypothyroidism. *Note: Goiter is absent if the cause of the hypothyroidism is secondary hypothyroidism from TSH deficiency since there is nothing in that condition to stimulate thyroid growth.*
- Hoarseness and voice changes if the enlarged thyroid presses on the vocal cords
- Facial and periorbital puffiness may occur from deposition of hyaluronic acid with non-pitting swelling (*myxedema*) in the connective tissues of the face and around the eyes. There may also be non-pitting edema in the hands and lower legs and feet, all a consequence of severe deficiency in thyroid hormone. The non-pitting edema of hypothyroidism is more widespread than the non-pitting edema of hyperthyroidism, which is more specific to the lower legs and is believed due to an autoimmune process.
- Joint and muscle pain from reduced muscle metabolism, weakness, and fatigue
- Sluggish tendon reflexes from slowed nerve conduction and motor neuron excitability
- Pleural and pericardial effusions from reduced cardiac output
- Carpal tunnel syndrome in hypothyroidism may have to do with fluid retention, reduced nerve conduction, and/or myxedematous hyaluronic acid deposits in the soft tissues around the wrist.
- Sensorineural hearing loss for which the mechanism is unclear. Thyroid hormone is important for the development and function of the auditory system.
- Hypoventilation from depressed respiratory drive and respiratory muscle weakness
- *Myxedema coma* (the extreme end of the spectrum of hypothyroidism, usually from discontinuing thyroid hormone replacement)

Causes of Hypothyroidism

Hypothyroidism is the undersecretion of thyroid hormone, for which there are various possible causes:

- *Hashimoto's Thyroiditis*, an autoimmune disease manifest as a lymphocytic infiltration of the thyroid, may cause hyperthyroidism at first due to a leak of stored thyroid hormones into the bloodstream ("*Hashitoxicosis*"). Over time, though, hypothyroidism sets in as autoimmunity continues to destroy thyroid tissue. In developed countries Hashimoto thyroiditis is the most common cause of thyroid enlargement. In underdeveloped countries it is iodine deficiency.

- *Iodine deficiency* (does not allow thyroid hormone to be produced)
- *Thyroid surgery* or *RAI treatment*
- Medications: *Cortisol* feedback to the pituitary gland inhibits not only adrenocorticotropic hormone (ACTH) secretion, but TSH secretion, as well as other pituitary hormones. *Amiodarone*, used to treat arrhythmias, has a lot of **iod**ine, which can interfere with thyroid hormone synthesis. *Lithium*, used as a mood stabilizer in bipolar disorder, can inhibit the release of thyroid hormone.
- *Congenital hypothyroidism* (often genetic)
- Hypothalamic or pituitary dysfunction, including tumors, surgery, radiation, bleeding (e.g., *Sheehan syndrome* – post-partum pituitary gland necrosis), infiltrative disease (*hemochromatosis*, *sarcoidosis*), and genetic disorders of the hypothalamus or pituitary gland can cause a deficiency in thyroid-stimulating hormone.
- In *thyroid hormone resistance syndrome*, there is decreased tissue sensitivity to thyroid hormone, effectively reducing the effect of thyroid hormone.
- Rare tumors may produce a thyroid hormone inactivating enzyme, *type 3 iodothyronine deiodinase*.

Diagnosis of Hypothyroidism

Apart from the history and physical examination, some tests are more specific in establishing the diagnosis of hypothyroidism and what might be causing it:

- *Free* thyroxine levels are low in hypothyroidism.
- Thyroid-stimulating hormone (TSH) levels are usually elevated in primary hypothyroidism as a response to low thyroid hormone. TSH may be low in secondary hypothyroidism secondary to pituitary dysfunction (**Fig. 3-2**).
- Antibody tests can check for anti-thyroid antibodies (e.g., thyroid peroxidase antibodies or thyroglobulin antibodies in Hashimoto's thyroiditis).
- Imaging. Ultrasound, CT scan, and MRI can assess the size and shape of abnormalities in the thyroid or pituitary gland.
- **TRH stimulation test**. If TSH does not rise following administering thyroid-releasing hormone (TRH, secreted by the hypothalamus), this may indicate a pituitary inability to secrete TSH.
- Acute-phase reactants, e.g., erythrocyte sedimentation rate (ESR) and C-reactive protein (CRP) may be used to assess the level of inflammation in cases of inflammatory thyroiditis.
- Genetic testing may be done if a genetic cause is suspected.

Treatment of Hypothyroidism

The treatment of hypothyroidism is usually lifelong thyroid hormone replacement. This may include oral levothyroxine, a synthetic form of T4 (which is preferred to T3 because of its longer half-life), or natural desiccated animal thyroid (which is less commonly used due to the availability and standard dosing of synthetic thyroid hormone). Medications that may cause hypothyroidism, such as cortisol, lithium or amiodarone should be discontinued if feasible.

Goiter

A goiter can occur in either hyperthyroidism or hypothyroidism, but for different reasons. In *hyperthyroidism*, goiter results from constant overactivity of the thyroid gland in churning out thyroid hormones. In *hypothyroidism*, goiter may arise from high levels of TSH that constantly try to stimulate the underactive thyroid gland. Where there is an iodine-deficient diet, goiter may arise as a compensatory response, with the thyroid attempting to capture more iodine from the bloodstream. In Hashimoto's thyroiditis, an autoimmune disorder, chronic inflammation of the thyroid may be responsible. There are also rare genetic mutations in which TSH receptor mutations cause increased sensitivity of the thyroid gland to TSH, resulting in excessive growth and enlargement of the thyroid gland. Not all cases of hyperthyroidism and hypothyroidism, though, lead to goiter formation.

Thyroiditis

Thyroiditis can occur in several forms:

- **Hashimoto's thyroiditis (chronic autoimmune thyroiditis)** is usually painless. The thyroid may have a diffusely enlarged, firm, and rubbery feel, but in some cases may be normal or even reduced in size due to the progressive destruction of thyroid tissue. Hashimoto's may at first be manifest as hyperthyroidism, but later as hypothyroidism, at which time it is treated with thyroid hormone replacement.
  People with one autoimmune disorder, like type 1 diabetes, have a higher likelihood of developing another

autoimmune disorder. Hashimoto's thyroiditis and Graves' disease are autoimmune thyroid disorders that are more common in people with type 1 diabetes.

- **Acute thyroiditis** (usually painful) may be bacterial with local abscess formation. It may initially be associated with hyperthyroidism, but later, when the inflammation damages the thyroid gland, may lead to hypothyroidism. It can be treated with antibiotics and pain medication.
- **Subacute thyroiditis** (**deQuervain's thyroiditis**) is believed to be viral in origin. The gland may at first feel tender and swollen but this may later subside, leaving a painless goiter. When tender, it may be treated with anti-inflammatory drugs and sometimes short-term corticosteroids.
- **Silent thyroiditis (painless thyroiditis)**, believed due to an autoimmune process, may cause transitory hyperthyroidism followed by a period of hypothyroidism, with later return of thyroid function to normal. The transient hyperthyroidism may be treated with beta-blockers to provide relief from the uncomfortable cardiovascular symptoms of hyperthyroidism.
- **Post-partum thyroiditis** (typically painless) occurs in the first year after childbirth and is believed to be autoimmune in origin. It starts with a hyperthyroid phase, followed by a hypothyroid phase, often returning to normal with 6-12 months.
- **Reidel's thyroiditis**, which may be painful due to inflammation and fibrosis, is a rare thyroiditis characterized by progressive fibrosis of the thyroid gland. It may cause hyperthyroidism in its early inflammatory state, and hypothyroidism when the thyroid tissue becomes replaced by fibrous tissue. Management may include pain relief medication, steroids, or surgery to relieve compressive symptoms, such as difficulty swallowing or breathing.

Thyroid Cancer

Most thyroid nodules are benign, but about 5-15% are malignant. Thyroid cancer may not have any noticeable symptoms at first and is often discovered on routine physical exam or imaging tests done for other reasons. Eventually, certain signs commonly appear:

- A lump in the neck, usually painless. A painful lump is most likely due to hemorrhage into a thyroid cyst.
- Enlargement of the thyroid gland
- Hoarseness, when the tumor is near the vocal cords
- Difficulty swallowing or breathing when the tumor impinges on the esophagus or trachea. There may by fixation of the nodule to nearby structures.
- Neck discomfort around the thyroid gland
- Nearby lymph node enlargement

Although thyroid cancers are commonly non-secretory or minimally-secretory, they need to be considered in thyroid evaluations. There are several kinds of thyroid cancer:

1. **Papillary thyroid cancer** is the most common, about 80% of thyroid cancers. It arises from thyroid follicle cells (the cells that produce thyroid hormone), grows slowly, and has a good prognosis.
2. **Follicular thyroid cancer** (about 10-15% of thyroid cancers) also originates from follicular cells. It is more common in areas with iodine deficiency. It has a higher chance of metastasis than does the papillary kind.
3. **Medullary thyroid cancer** (about 5-10% of thyroid cancers) arises from parafollicular cells (*C cells*), which produce calcitonin. In some cases, medullary thyroid cancer is hereditary. Calcitonin levels are often elevated, aiding the diagnosis. The prognosis depends largely on its stage.
4. **Anaplastic thyroid cancer** is rare (< 2%) but aggressive. It arises from cells derived from follicular thyroid cells, grows fast, spreads extensively, and has a poor prognosis.
5. **Thyroid lymphoma** (rare) arises from lymphocytes. It may occur in people with a pre-existing autoimmune thyroid disease, e.g., Hashimoto's thyroiditis. It has a variable prognosis, depending on its type, stage, patient's overall health and age, and how well it responds to treatment.
6. **Hürthle cell carcinoma**, a rare type, often more aggressive than other thyroid cancers, arises from thyroid *Hürthle (oxyphil) cells*, a uniquely appearing type of follicular cell that produces thyroid hormone, like other follicular cells.

The diagnosis of thyroid cancer is made through a combination of history and exam, imaging tests (e.g., ultrasound, CT, MRI, PET scan, RAI scan), tumor markers (e.g., elevated calcitonin in medullary thyroid cancer; increasing thyroglobulin that may suggest the recurrence of papillary or follicular thyroid cancer), and biopsy. Hot nodules on scan have a decreased risk of malignancy, as do cysts. The treatment, depending on the type of cancer and stage, may involve thyroidectomy, lymph node dissection, radioactive iodine therapy, external beam radiation, chemotherapy, and/or hormone replacement.

Euthyroid Sick Syndrome

It is possible to have abnormal thyroid tests and a normally functioning thyroid gland. In **euthyroid sick syndrome (non-thyroidal illness syndrome; NTIS)**, abnormal thyroid function test results can appear but the thyroid gland itself is functioning normally (euthyroid). Euthyroid sick syndrome is commonly observed in critically ill patients, those with severe infections, major surgery, trauma, burns, and other critical medical conditions. There are several possible reasons for NTIS:

- Decreased T3 levels in euthyroid sick patients may partly be due to reduced conversion of T4 (thyroxine) to T3 in peripheral tissue.
- Decreased thyroid binding globulin (TBG) levels can decrease total T4 and T3 levels without affecting the free fractions.
- Some drugs can interfere with the binding of thyroid hormone to its carrier proteins (e.g., furosemide, NSAIDs).
- Circulating antibodies can sometimes interfere with the laboratory assay.

It is important to differentiate euthyroid sick syndrome from primary thyroid disorders, such as hypothyroidism or hyperthyroidism, as the management of these conditions differ. If a patient is suspected of euthyroid sick syndrome, treatment will focus on addressing the underlying illness rather than specific thyroid hormone replacement therapy. Euthyroid sick syndrome typically reverses with resolution of the underlying illness.

Calcitonin

The parafollicular (C cells) of the thyroid gland respond to high blood calcium by secreting calcitonin, which helps reduce blood calcium by inhibiting bone resorption (breakdown) by bone osteoclast cells, thus preventing excessive bone loss. This is opposite to the effect of parathyroid hormone (PTH), which stimulates osteoclast activity. The interplay between calcitonin and PTH helps maintain the balance of calcium in the body.

Calcitonin, though, has a relatively small influence on bones in comparison with PTH. It has been useful, though, as a tumor marker produced by medullary thyroid cancers that arise from C cells. It also has therapeutic uses as an inhibitor of osteoclastic bone resorption.

Chapter 4 Parathyroid Glands

Four parathyroid glands lie behind the thyroid gland (**Fig. 4-1**). They produce **parathyroid hormone (PTH)** and also a small amount **of parathyroid hormone-related protein** (**PTHrP**).

Parathyroid Hormone (PTH)

Parathyroid hormone (PTH) is important in regulating calcium and phosphate levels in the blood. Calcium is important for:

- Bone health, being an important component of bone
- Muscle contraction of both skeletal and smooth muscle
- Nerve function (in transmitting nerve impulses)
- Blood clotting
- Enzyme activation
- Hormone regulation (via PTH and calcitonin)

PTH raises blood calcium when needed by:

- Increasing *calcium reabsorption* and *phosphate excretion* in the *kidneys*. This results in increased blood calcium and lower blood phosphate.
- Enhancing *bone* breakdown (*resorption*) to release calcium and phosphate into the bloodstream.
- Stimulating the activation of vitamin D in the kidney; vitamin D enhances the absorption of calcium and phosphate from the *intestines* and reabsorption of calcium and phosphate from the *kidneys* (**Fig. 4-1**).

Calcitonin has the opposite effect of PTH, but PTH and vitamin D have a more significant impact on blood calcium.

Hyperparathyroidism

There are three main types of hyperparathyroidism, all of which can cause hypercalcemia:

1. In **primary hyperparathyroidism** (the most common type), the main problem lies in the parathyroid gland. There is an enlargement or overactivity of *one or more* parathyroid glands, causing excess production of parathyroid hormone (PTH) and elevated blood calcium levels. This may lead to kidney stones, osteoporosis, and other symptoms (**Fig. 4-3**). Usually, the excess PTH is due to a benign secreting tumor (*parathyroid adenoma*). Sometimes there may be multiple parathyroid adenomas, parathyroid hyperplasia, or, rarely, a parathyroid carcinoma that secretes excess amounts of PTH. There are also rare non-parathyroid PTH-secreting tumors.
2. **Secondary hyperparathyroidism** is commonly a compensatory response of PTH secretion to something that causes low calcium or high phosphate levels in the blood. The diet may be exceptionally low in calcium, or there may be malabsorption of calcium and vitamin D, as in celiac disease, inflammatory bowel disease, or gastric bypass. The kidneys in chronic kidney

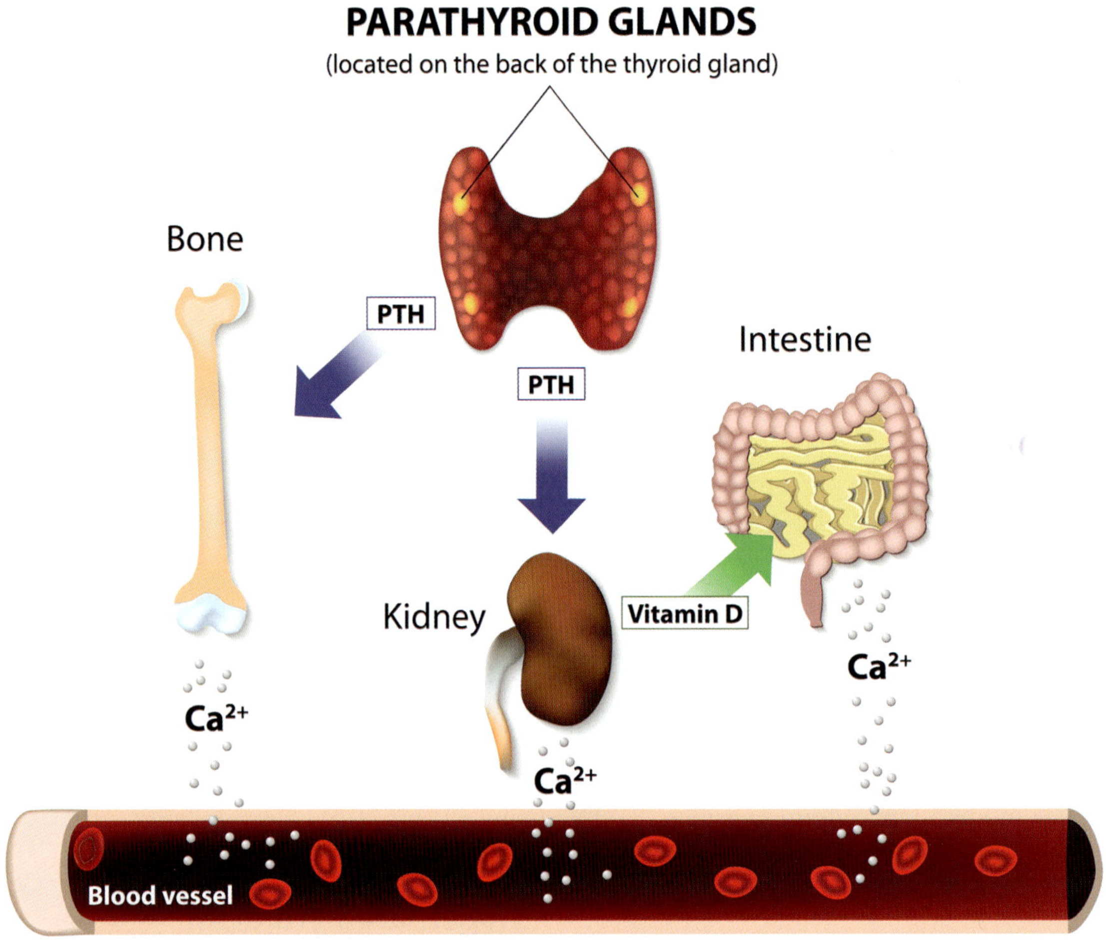

Fig. 4-1. Effects of parathyroid hormone on calcium and vitamin D.

disease may have difficulty activating vitamin D or excreting phosphate. Certain anticonvulsants (*dilantin, phenobarbital*) can decrease the levels of vitamin D.

There may also be a malfunctioning of the calcium-sensing receptors (CaSR) on parathyroid and kidney cells (lithium can do this; the condition may also be familial). If the CaSR doesn't respond to calcium, the parathyroid gland and kidney *think* that calcium is low, so the parathyroid gland oversecretes PTH and the kidney overabsorbs calcium to try to restore normal calcium levels. This results in *hypocalciuric hypercalcemia* (**Fig. 4-2**). Conversely, if the CaSR is *oversensitive* to calcium, another inherited condition, the parathyroid gland and kidney think there is too much calcium and won't reabsorb it in the kidney or secrete PTH, leading to increased calcium excretion and hypocalcemia (*hypercalciuric hypocalcemia*) (**Fig. 4-2**).

Secondary hyperparathyroidism is typically characterized by an increase in the size and activity of *all* the parathyroid glands.

3. **Tertiary hyperparathyroidism** occurs when secondary hyperparathyroidism persists and becomes autonomous. I.e., the overactive parathyroid glands no longer respond to normal feedback mechanisms. In tertiary hyperparathyroidism, one or more of the parathyroids becomes continuously overactive (which can happen with long-standing kidney disease or after kidney transplantation) even after the cause of secondary hyperparathyroidism has been corrected.

The **diagnosis of hyperparathyroidism**, apart from the symptoms and signs of hypercalcemia (**Fig. 4-3**), may involve:

- Blood tests for the levels of calcium (elevated), PTH (elevated), phosphate (low, since PTH causes the excretion of phosphate), vitamin D (may be low, normal, or high) and kidney function tests (a kidney problem might lead to reduced vitamin D production)
- Urine test for 24-hour calcium excretion (elevated due to high blood levels of calcium)

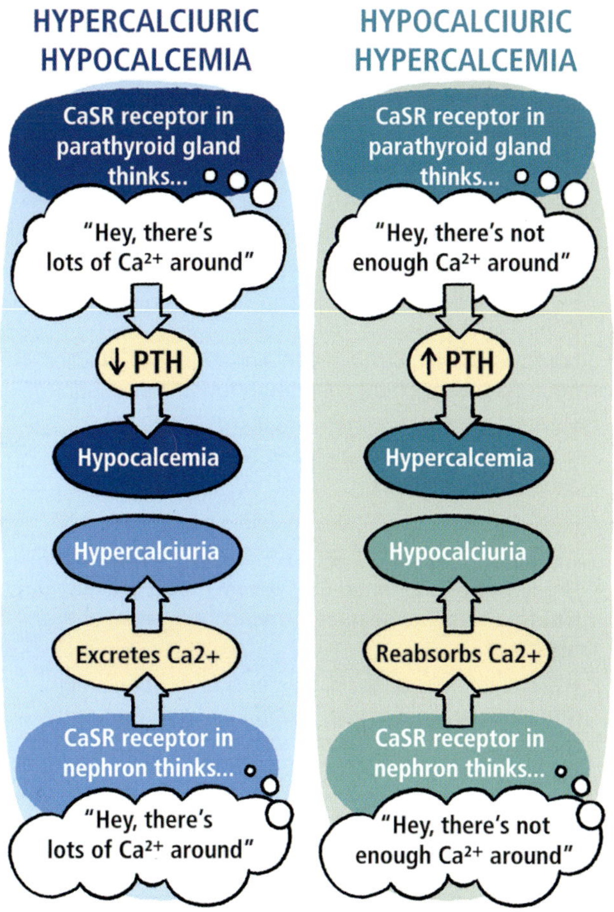

Fig. 4-2. Modified from Berkowitz, A. Clinical Pathophysiology Made Ridiculously Simple. Medmaster.

- Imaging studies of the parathyroid glands with ultrasound, CT, or MRI. In a *sestamibi scan*, radioactive technetium-99m sestamibi, which has an affinity for parathyroid tissue, is absorbed by the overactive parathyroid gland and detected by a SPECT scanner, helping to identify which parathyroid gland is involved and where the abnormal gland may be, whether in the thyroid or other area of the neck or even thorax. (The test frequently has a false negative result, so other tests may be needed, too). A bone scan may also help in assessing the clinical impact of the disease.
- Genetic testing as clinically indicated

The **treatment of primary hyperparathyroidism** may include:

- Simply observing when symptoms are mild, monitoring calcium levels and renal function
- Parathyroidectomy for symptomatic patients with kidney stones or osteoporosis. Radiation therapy may be considered when surgery is not an option.
- Medications:
  - Phosphate binders (reduce the levels of the phosphate that stimulates PTH secretion); restriction of dietary phosphate
  - Vitamin D analogs (if vitamin D is low) to maintain bone health
  - Calcimimetics. *Cinacalcet*, a calcimimetic, reduces the secretion of parathyroid hormone by binding to and activating calcium-sensing receptors on parathyroid cells and tricking them into thinking blood calcium levels are higher than they are. This decreases PTH secretion.
  - *Bisphosphonates* help decrease bone loss by inhibiting osteoclasts and reduce the risk of fractures associated with osteoporosis. *Denosumab* is a monoclonal antibody medication that inhibits bone breakdown by inhibiting the activity of osteoclasts.
- Lifestyle and diet. Avoiding excessive calcium intake, hydration to prevent kidney stones, and regular exercise

The **treatment of secondary hyperparathyroidism** includes:

- Treating the underlying cause (e.g., kidney dysfunction, malabsorption of vitamin D and calcium)
- Vitamin D and calcium supplements
- Phosphate binders to reduce phosphate levels; restriction of dietary phosphate
- Calcimimetics to reduce PTH secretion
- Dialysis if needed in end-stage renal disease to manage calcium and phosphate levels

Treating tertiary hyperparathyroidism involves surgical removal of the persistently hyperactive parathyroid glands.

Hypoparathyroidism

Hypoparathyroidism may occur with surgical removal of the parathyroid glands or radiation therapy to the parathyroid glands, causing hypocalcemia. It may also be due to autoimmune destruction of the parathyroid glands, or to genetic conditions marked by underactivity of the parathyroid glands (e.g., **DeGeorge syndrome**, **Kenny-Caffey syndrome** and others) or idiopathic. Severe magnesium deficiency can also do it, since magnesium is needed for proper functioning of the parathyroid glands.

Pseudohypoparathyrodism (PHP) Type 1a (**Albright hereditary osteodystrophy**) is an autosomal dominant genetic disorder with *resistance to the actions of PTH* (and sometimes to thyroid-stimulating hormone or gonadotropins as well). It is called "pseudo" because the symptoms of hypocalcemia (**Fig. 4-4**) might suggest low parathyroid hormone levels, but the PTH level is actually higher than normal; the body just cannot respond to the PTH. The condition can include short stature, shortened hand bones (brachydactyly), subcutaneous ossification, and developmental delay. **Pseudohypoparathyroidism Type 1b** resembles PHP type 1a, but without the abnormal physical features.

Treatment of pseudohypoparathyroidism includes calcium and vitamin D supplements.

Pseudopseudohypoparathyroidism (PPHP) is caused by autosomal dominant mutations to the same gene as PHP and can have similar skeletal abnormalities (Albright's hereditary osteodystrophy), but differs in having normal calcium and PTH levels, and no resistance to PTH.

I am unaware of a condition called pseudo-pseudopseudohypoparathyroidism.

Hypercalcemia

The signs and symptoms of hyperparathyroidism and hypoparathyroidism often parallel those of hypercalcemia and hypocalcemia, as described in **Figures 4-3** and **4-4**.

FIGURE 4-3. SYMPTOMS AND SIGNS OF HYPERCALCEMIA

Stones, Bones, abdominal *Groans,* psychiatric *Moans:*

- Kidney *stones*
- *Bone* pain and osteoporosis (when the hypercalcemia is due to bone breakdown)
- *Digestive* symptoms, e.g., nausea and vomiting, loss of appetite, abdominal pain, constipation. (Hypercalcemia can slow gut motility.)
- *Lethargy, depression, personality change, and confusion.* (High calcium can slow signal conduction in neurons and interfere with neurotransmitter release.)
- Increased thirst, frequent urination, dehydration. (Excess calcium excretion can be accompanied by excess water loss.)
- Hypertension. (High calcium levels can lead to vasoconstriction and increased cardiac contractility.)
- Bradycardia, shortened QT interval. (High calcium can interfere with the electrical conduction system of the heart.)
- Hyperchloremic acidosis. (Hypercalcemia can cause renal tubular dysfunction, leading to decreased renal reabsorption of bicarbonate, with compensatory retention of blood chloride.)
- Muscle weakness (proximal myopathy), twitches. (Calcium plays a key role in muscle contraction.)
- Calcific band keratopathy (calcium deposits in the cornea)

Causes of Hypercalcemia

Hypercalcemia can have a variety of causes:

- **Increased Intestinal Absorption of Calcium** may occur with hyperparathyroidism or with excess vitamin D or calcium in the diet. *Milk-alkali syndrome* is a metabolic alkalosis combined with hypercalcemia and renal impairment that results from ingesting large amounts of calcium and alkali, often through calcium-containing antacids.
- **Increased Bone Resorption (breakdown)** with release of calcium can occur with hyperparathyroidism, with a non-parathyroid PTH-secreting tumor, tumor metastasis to bone, Paget's disease of bone, or prolonged bed rest. About 99% of total body calcium lies in the skeleton. Hyperthyroidism can increase bone turnover and raise blood calcium by stimulating bone osteoclasts.
- **Increased Kidney Reabsorption of Calcium** occurs in hyperparathyroidism through excess PTH secretion. It can also occur through excess vitamin D activation, which may sometimes occur in certain granulomatous diseases (sarcoid, tuberculosis). Granulomas are clusters of immune cells that can produce calcitriol, the active form of vitamin D. Thiazide diuretics can also increase calcium reabsorption.

Diagnosis of Hypercalcemia

The origin of a hypercalcemia can be verified through the measurement of parathyroid hormone, vitamin D, calcitonin levels, kidney function tests, markers of bone metabolism (e.g., alkaline phosphatase), and imaging studies.

Treatment for Hypercalcemia

Treatment for hypercalcemia can include:

- Hydration (to dilute blood calcium and promote excretion of excess calcium through the kidneys)
- Medications:
  - Biphosphonates (e.g., *zoledronic acid, pamidronate*) inhibit bone breakdown and lower blood calcium levels.
  - Calcitonin (lowers blood calcium)
  - Glucocorticoids can reduce the inflammation associated with certain causes of hypercalcemia, and can reduce the activation of vitamin D.

- *Denosumab* inhibits osteoclasts and is used in certain malignancies that have hypercalcemia.
- *Cinacalcet* is a calcimimetic that reduces PTH levels by increasing the sensitivity of the Calcium-Sensing Receptor (CaSR) in the parathyroid glands to calcium, causing the receptor to think there is too much calcium.
- Surgery can remove a parathyroid adenoma in primary hyperparathyroidism or treat an underlying malignancy that is causing hypercalcemia.
- Dialysis can remove excess calcium from the blood.

Hypocalcemia

Figure 4-4 describes the main symptoms and signs of hypocalcemia.

Causes of Hypocalcemia

The main causes of hypocalcemia include:

- Hypoparathyroidism (surgical, autoimmune, familial / genetic, or idiopathic)
- *Pseudohypoparathyroidism* (resistance to PTH)

FIGURE 4-4. SIGNS & SYMPTOMS OF HYPOCALCEMIA
• **Tingling and Numbness**: Often felt in the fingertips, toes, and around the mouth
• **Muscle Cramps and Spasms**: Particularly in the hands and feet
• **Tetany**: Involuntary contraction of muscles, which may lead to muscle stiffness or spasms. Tetany can also occur with hypomagnesemia and alkalosis.
• **Seizures**: In severe cases, hypocalcemia can cause epileptic seizures.
• **Chvostek's Sign**: Tapping on the facial nerve triggers twitching of the facial muscles.
• **Trousseau's Sign**: Inflating a blood pressure cuff on the arm induces carpal spasm.
• **Arrhythmias**: Abnormal heart rhythms
• **Hypotension**: From decreased strength of cardiac contraction and dilation of peripheral blood vessels
• **Heart Failure**: In severe, acute cases, hypocalcemia can lead to heart failure.
• **Confusion, Depression, Anxiety**
• **Dry Skin and Brittle Nails**: Chronic hypocalcemia can affect skin and nail health.
• **Eye Problems**: Cataracts can develop in chronic cases.
• **Dental Problems**: In children, chronic hypocalcemia can lead to delayed formation of teeth and enamel defects.

- Vitamin D deficiency
- Low dietary calcium
- Kidney dysfunction
- Medications: Loop diuretics (e.g., furosemide), bisphosphonates (e.g., *zoledronic acid, pamidronate*), calcitonin, some anticonvulsants (e.g., phenytoin), and some chemotherapy drugs can cause hypocalcemia.
- Acute pancreatitis can release enzymes that cause fat necrosis; calcium binds to the free fatty acids.
- Malabsorption syndromes can interfere with calcium absorption.
- Hypoalbuminemia. Albumin binds to calcium. Reduced albumin lowers the level of total calcium, while the level of ionized calcium (the biologically active form) may be normal. It is therefore important to measure *ionized* calcium to determine the degree of *functional* calcium loss.
- Hyperphosphatemia. High blood levels of phosphate can bind to calcium, reducing the amount of available ionized calcium.
- Magnesium deficiency or excess can decrease PTH secretion and action.
- Acute citrate toxicity. (Citrate binds to calcium.)
- Post-surgical hypoparathyroidism (following thyroid or parathyroid surgery)
- Certain genetic disorders:
    - Vitamin D resistance
    - Reduced production or impaired response to PTH
    - Underdevelopment of the parathyroid glands
    - *Autosomal Dominant Hypocalcemia*. An over-sensitive calcium-sensing receptor causes inadequate secretion of PTH.
- Certain critical illnesses that involve electrolyte imbalances
- *Elevated calcitonin is not a significant cause of hypocalcemia, since the effect of calcitonin is minor in comparison with parathyroid hormone, vitamin D, or kidney function.*

Diagnosis of Hypocalcemia

The determination of the cause of hypocalcemia includes:

- Blood tests:
    - Directly measure ionized calcium (the active form). Or, measure total serum calcium, in which an adjustment is made depending on albumin levels.
    - Blood levels of parathyroid hormone, vitamin D, phosphate, and magnesium
- Kidney function tests
- Imaging to evaluate the parathyroid glands if a parathyroid disorder is suspected. In chronic

hypoparathyroidism, imaging may show calcifications in the basal ganglia of the brain due to the binding of high phosphate with calcium.

Treatment of Hypocalcemia

Treatment of hypocalcemia may include:

- Calcium supplementation (e.g., calcium carbonate; calcium citrate)
- Vitamin D supplementation, including sunlight exposure
- Intravenous calcium
- Correcting the underlying cause (e.g., hypoparathyroidism, kidney dysfunction)
- Adjusting medications that might cause hypocalcemia (certain diuretics, antiepileptic drugs)
- Dietary modification to increase calcium intake (dairy products, leafy green vegetables, fortified foods)
- In some cases, treatment with PTH. (*Teriparatide* is a form of parathyroid hormone.)

Hungry Bone Syndrome

Hungry bone syndrome (HBS) is a complication that can occur after parathyroid surgery, particularly in patients with hyperparathyroidism or other conditions that cause elevated parathyroid hormone (PTH) levels. The syndrome is characterized by a sudden drop in PTH levels following surgery, leading to a significant uptake of calcium and other minerals by the bones. The bones become "hungry" for minerals, and this can lead to hypocalcemia, hypophosphatemia, and hypomagnesemia.

The rapid uptake of minerals by bones can cause bone pain, and in rare cases, it can lead to fractures, particularly in patients with weakened bones due to long-standing hyperparathyroidism. Hungry bone syndrome can also affect the heart, leading to irregular heart rhythms and other cardiac issues.

Note that not all patients who undergo parathyroid surgery will develop hungry bone syndrome. The risk of this condition is higher in patients who have very high PTH levels before surgery.

Parathyroid Hormone-Related Protein (PTHrP)

PTHrP shares certain structural and function similarities with parathyroid hormone (PTH) but is produced by different tissues throughout the body, not just the parathyroid glands (e.g., placenta, breast, lung, kidney, skin). It also has more widespread functions, apart from calcium and phosphate regulation. In the placenta, it helps to transfer calcium from the mother to the developing fetus, is involved in the development of the mammary glands during pregnancy and contributes to lactation by promoting milk secretion. PTHrP also helps regulate bone formation and growth. In adults, it is involved with bone remodeling and repair.

PTHrP can be overproduced by certain malignant and non-malignant tumors of the lung, breast, kidney, ovary, and other tissues and contribute to hypercalcemia. Prolonged bed rest and excess vitamin D can also result in elevated PTHrP and hypercalcemia.

The diagnosis of excess PTHrP can be made with a blood test to measure PTHrP concentration, in conjunction with calcium, phosphate, and PTH levels. Imaging studies (CT, MRI, PET scans) can be used to help identify tumors.

Treatment of excess PTHrP depends on the cause:

- Treat the tumor if it exists (e.g., surgery, radiation, chemotherapy, targeted therapies, immunotherapy).
- The hypercalcemia of immobilization can be treated with increased physical activity and adequate hydration to maintain calcium levels.
- *Bisphosphonates* (e.g., *alendronate, risedronate, pamidronate, zoledronic acid*) reduce bone breakdown.
- *Calcitonin* inhibits osteoclast activity and increases urinary calcium excretion.
- *Denosumab* is a monoclonal antibody that inhibits one of the proteins used in bone remodeling, reducing the release of calcium from the bones.
- *Corticosteroids* reduce the gut's absorption of calcium and decrease the conversion of vitamin D to its active form, calcitriol, in the kidneys.

Vitamin D

While vitamin D is well-known as a dietary source (fatty fish, egg yolks, and fortified foods like milk and breakfast cereals), and as a vitamin supplement, it is also a hormone produced in the skin in response to sunlight (ultraviolet radiation). Vitamin D plays essential roles in the body:

- Vitamin D in its active form, *calcitriol* (1,25-dihydroxyvitamin D3), promotes calcium and phosphorus absorption from the intestines (as does PTH) and kidneys (although PTH promotes phosphorus *loss* in the kidneys).
- Bone health: Vitamin D promotes the deposition of calcium and phosphorus into bone. In certain circumstances, though, when blood calcium is low, PTH secretion increases and causes the

increased production of vitamin D, which, at the higher concentration, can *stimulate* bone osteoclastic bone breakdown and promote the release of calcium from bone, to bring blood calcium levels back up to normal.

- Both PTH and vitamin D, at low levels, increase bone building, but at high levels promote bone breakdown. It is a complex relationship that also depends on the concentration of calcium and phosphate in the blood at the time. Both vitamin D and PTH help maintain proper density and mineralization of bones by calcium and phosphate.
- Immune system: Vitamin D can reduce inflammation by decreasing the production of pro-inflammatory cytokines.
- Tissue development: Vitamin D can inhibit excess cell proliferation and promote cell differentiation.
- Muscle function: Vitamin D supplementation when vitamin D levels are low can improve muscle strength and function.
- Cardiovascular health: Vitamin D is involved in lowering blood pressure, partly by suppressing the activity of the renin-angiotensin-aldosterone system; it helps regulate blood clotting and maintain the normal function of cardiac muscle cells.
- Brain health: Vitamin D receptors are found in many brain areas. Vitamin D may play a role in neurodevelopment and neurotransmitter regulation and improve cognition.

Vitamin D Synthesis

The synthesis of active vitamin D occurs in several steps (**Fig. 4-5**):

- Vitamin D synthesis starts when the skin is exposed to sunlight and synthesizes vitamin

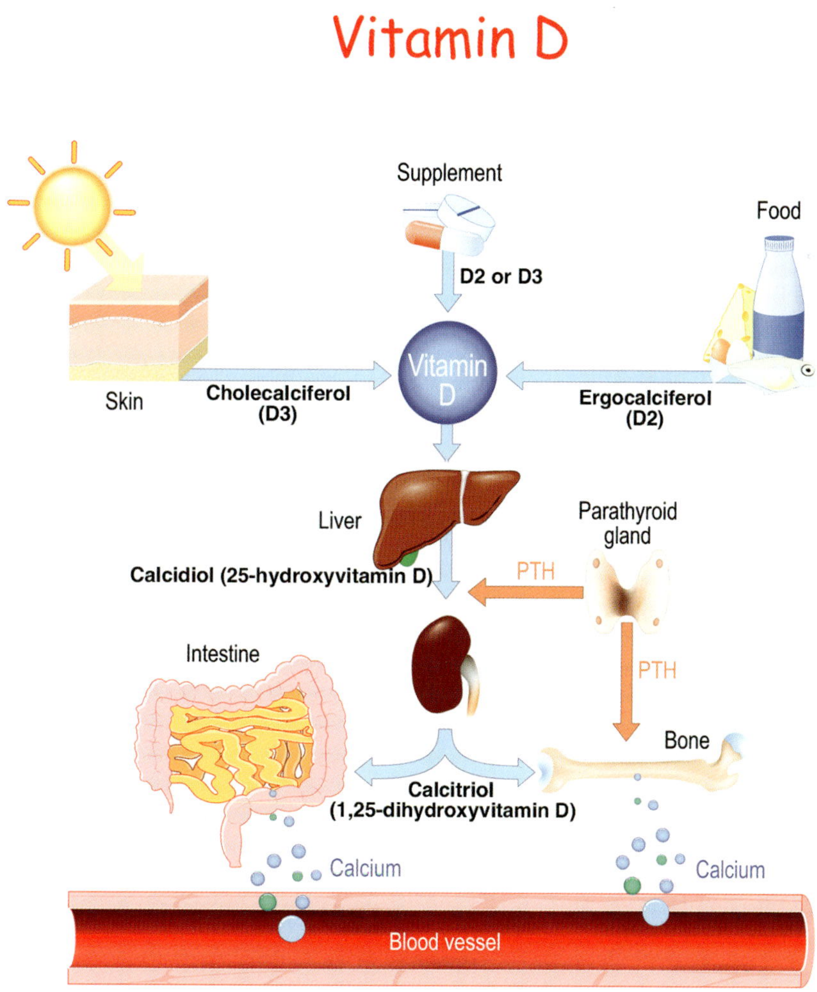

Fig. 4-5. Vitamin D synthesis.

D3 (*cholecalciferol*) or the body ingests vitamin D in the form of vitamin D3 or D2 (*ergocalciferol,* obtained mainly in the diet, not the skin).

- D3 and D2 are inactive and change in the *liver,* where D3 is converted to 25-hydroxyvitamin D3 (*calcifediol; calcidiol*) and vitamin D2 is converted to 25-hydroxyvitamin D2.
- Next, the *kidney,* under the influence of parathyroid hormone, converts 25-hydroxyvitamin D3 to 1,25-dihydroxyvitamin D3 (*calcitriol*), and 25-hydroxyvitamin D2 to 1,25-dihydroxyvitamin D2. Of these, calcitriol (the D3 form) is the most active form of vitamin D.

Hypervitaminosis D

Too much vitamin D in the blood can arise from taking an excess of vitamin D supplements. It can also occur in hyperparathyroidism, since parathyroid hormone increases the production of active vitamin D in the kidney. Certain granulomatous diseases (sarcoid, Tb, histoplasmosis) can cause an increase in active vitamin D, as granulomatous macrophages can produce the enzyme *1-alpha-hydroxylase,* which converts inactive vitamin D to its active form. The result of all of these is hypercalcemia, for which the symptoms and signs are described in **Figure 4-3**.

The diagnosis of hypervitaminosis D can be made by measuring serum levels of 25-hydroxyvitamin D (the main circulating form of vitamin D), as well as calcium, phosphate, and PTH levels. PTH levels may be decreased due to PTH suppression by the high blood calcium levels. Imaging studies (bone densitometry, skeletal X-rays) may help, as high levels of vitamin D can lead to bone resorption, with reduced bone density and increased fracture risk. Imaging studies can be used to follow the patient after treatment, which largely consists of discontinuing vitamin D supplements and addressing hydration and GI issues, as well as underlying medical conditions (excess sun exposure, tumors, diseases that change vitamin D to its active form).

Hypovitaminosis D

The symptoms and signs of vitamin D deficiency include:

- Hypocalcemia
- Bone and muscle pain. (Vitamin D helps prevent osteomalacia and rickets and appears to play a role in muscle function as well.)
- Increased susceptibility to infections, and impaired wound healing. (Vitamin D helps regulate the body's immune responses and can stimulate the production of antimicrobial peptides.)
- Mood disorders. (There are vitamin D receptors in many areas of the brain, and they may play a role in brain function, including the production of certain neurotransmitters.)
- Hair loss. (Hair follicles have vitamin D receptors, which may play a role in the cycle of hair growth and shedding.)
- Rickets (in children) or osteomalacia (in adults) due to impaired bone mineralization
- Osteoporosis from increased bone resorption. Ingesting too much vitamin A can also cause osteoporosis. It has been proposed that excess vitamin A represses osteoblasts and stimulates osteoclasts, or that it may interfere with vitamin D metabolism.

Vitamin D deficiency can arise in several ways:

- Dietary intake of vitamin D may be inadequate.
- Malabsorption can affect the absorption of dietary fats, and vitamin D is a fat-soluble vitamin.
- Chronic pancreatitis can cause exocrine pancreatic insufficiency with a deficit in enzymes to break down fat for vitamin D absorption.
- Chronic kidney disease and chronic liver disease can impair vitamin D synthesis.
- Inadequate sun exposure
- Inflammatory bowel disease can decrease the area available for vitamin D absorption.
- Some anticonvulsants and antifungals can inhibit the change of vitamin D to its active form.
- Certain genetic disorders may affect the synthesis or absorption of vitamin D or make the body resistant to it.
- Melanin in the skin can reduce the skin's capacity to produce vitamin D3. Pigmented individuals are at greater risk of developing vitamin D deficiency.

Vitamin D deficiency can be diagnosed through measurement of serum levels of 25-hydroxyvitamin D, imaging (X-rays, bone densitometry for osteoporosis), calcium, phosphate, magnesium, alkaline phosphate, creatinine (for kidney function), and PTH levels. (PTH may be high in response to the hypocalcemia.)

The **treatment** of vitamin D deficiency includes vitamin D supplements, adequate sun exposure, nutritional modification (foods rich in vitamin D: fatty fish, fortified dairy products, eggs, mushrooms exposed to ultraviolet light), and dealing with the underlying cause (e.g., malabsorption).

Rickets

Rickets is a disease of children. It is caused by a deficiency in vitamin D, calcium, or phosphate, which are needed for bone development and mineralization. The bones become soft, weak, and prone to deformities.

Kinds of rickets:

1. *Nutritional rickets* is caused by deficiency of vitamin D, calcium, or phosphate in the diet, or in children who have limited sun exposure, or impaired nutrient absorption.
2. *Vitamin D-dependent rickets type 1 and type 2* are rare genetic disorders with impaired activation or response to vitamin D, resulting in poor calcium and phosphate absorption and poor mineralization of bones.
3. *Hypophophatemic rickets* is caused by a genetic defect with decreased phosphate reabsorption by the kidneys. There is insufficient phosphate available for bone mineralization.

Diagnosis of Rickets

Several observations contribute to the diagnosis of rickets:

- Skeletal deformities (bowed legs, knock knees, pigeon chest [protrusion of the sternum], prominent forehead).
- Delayed growth and short stature
- Muscle weakness
- Dental problems: Delayed tooth eruption, poor enamel formation, increased risk of cavities
- Bone pain, especially in wrists, ankles, knees, or ribs
- Blood tests: Calcium and phosphate (low in classical vitamin D deficiency rickets), alkaline phosphatase (increased bone turnover causes higher blood levels of alkaline phosphatase), parathyroid hormone (might be high in response to low calcium levels); 25-hydroxyvitamin D (measures the level of vitamin D in the blood)
- X-rays of bone: Widening of the growth plates, bone deformities, bone areas of decreased mineralization, *Looser's zones* (areas of severe osteomalacia that appear as thin, radiolucent lines on X-ray, mimicking fractures – more common in osteomalacia than in rickets)
- Bone density scan to assess bone mineral density
- Genetic testing

Treatment of Rickets

- Vitamin D supplementation: Ergocalciferol (vitamin D2) or cholecalciferol (vitamin D3)
- Calcium carbonate (or calcium citrate) and phosphate supplementation
- Sun exposure
- Balanced diet rich in vitamin D, calcium, and phosphate (fatty fish, fortified dairy products, eggs, and green leafy vegetables)
- Regular follow-up

Osteomalacia

Osteomalacia is characterized by softened bones due to impaired mineralization. It is the adult counterpart of rickets. The difference is that rickets occurs in children whose bones are still growing and fail to mineralize properly, whereas in osteomalacia the bones lose their mineralization.

In certain cases of suspected osteomalacia, a bone biopsy can provide direct evidence of impaired mineralization. Blood calcium is commonly tested for in routine blood tests.

Part of the treatment of osteomalacia is the management of underlying conditions, such as kidney disease (impaired vitamin D activation) or malabsorption disorders. Osteomalacia is treated similarly to rickets with vitamin D and calcium supplementation.

Osteoporosis

Osteoporosis is characterized by decreased bone mass and structural deterioration of bone tissue that leads to increased bone fragility and fracture risk. There is an imbalance between bone breakdown (by osteoclasts) and bone formation (by osteoblasts). The risks for developing osteoporosis include:

- *Age*: Bone remodeling becomes less efficient with age.
- *Gender*: Women are at higher risk. Estrogen plays an important role in maintaining bone density; hence, postmenopausal women are at a higher risk for osteoporosis. Testosterone is also important in maintaining bone health and drops in men with age.
- *Race*: Caucasian and Asian individuals are at higher risk.
- *Family history* of osteoporosis
- *Small body frame*
- *Overactive thyroid, parathyroid, or adrenal glands*: Thyroid hormones increase the rate of bone turnover; adrenal glands produce cortisol, which increases bone breakdown by stimulating osteoclasts, and decreases bone formation by inhibiting osteoblasts.
- *Hyperprolactinemia* can cause osteoporosis by decreasing the level of sex hormones.
- *Chronic low calcium or vitamin D intake*, whether through diet or malabsorption
- Some *long-term medications*: E.g., glucocorticoids, some antiepileptic drugs (may alter vitamin D metabolism), and proton pump inhibitors (may decrease calcium absorption)
- *Sedentary lifestyle*
- *Excess alcohol*: Can enhance osteoclast activity and

impair osteoblasts, hinder calcium and vitamin D metabolism, and decrease estrogen in women and testosterone in men

- *Excess caffeine*: May increase calcium excretion
- *Excess tobacco use*: Possible decreased intestinal calcium absorption, reduced bone blood supply, reduced osteoblast activity and increased osteoclast activity; decreased levels of estrogen and testosterone
- *Medical conditions*: Rheumatoid arthritis (inflammation, inactivity, glucocorticoid therapy), lupus (glucocorticoid therapy, inflammation, inactivity, kidney disease), multiple myeloma (increased osteoclast and decreased osteoblast activity), and other conditions may be associated with osteoporosis.
- *Radiation* or *chemotherapy*

Bone density testing with dual-energy X-ray absorptiometry (DEXA) scans can help assess changes in bone density over time. A T-score (compares the patient's bone density with that of a young, healthy adult of the same sex) of -1.0 or above is considered normal; T-scores between -1.0 and -2.5 indicate osteopenia (low bone density), and T-scores of -2.5 or below indicate osteoporosis. Conventional x-rays are unreliable for detecting changes in bone mass, since 30% of bone must be lost before the changes show on x-ray.

Treatment of Osteoporosis

The treatment for osteoporosis aims to halt bone loss, improve bone density, and prevent fractures. Treatment options for osteoporosis include:

- **Bisphosphonates**: These are the most commonly prescribed medications for osteoporosis.
  - *Alendronate (Fosamax)*: Taken orally
  - *Risedronate (Actonel)*: Taken orally
  - *Ibandronate (Boniva)*: Can be taken orally or via intravenous (IV) infusion
  - *Zoledronic Acid (Reclast)*: Administered via IV

  Bisphosphonates work by inhibiting bone resorption.
- **Selective Estrogen Receptor Modulators (SERMs)**:
  - *Raloxifene (Evista)*: This medication mimics estrogen's beneficial effects on bone density in postmenopausal women, without some of the side effects associated with estrogen.
- **Parathyroid Hormone Analog**: *Teriparatide (Forteo)* and *abaloparatide (Tymlos)* are analogs of parathyroid hormone that help stimulate bone formation when injected intermittently. The intermittent nature of the treatment has an anabolic effect, rather than the catabolic effect on bone commonly attributed to continuously secreting parathyroid hormone.
- **Monoclonal Antibody**: *Denosumab (Prolia)* is a biologic drug that inhibits osteoclast formation, thus reducing bone resorption.
- **Hormone Replacement Therapy (HRT)**: *Estrogen*, primarily used for postmenopausal women, can help maintain bone density. However, it is used less frequently due to concerns about increased risks of cancer, heart disease, and blood clots.
- **Calcitonin** inhibits bone resorption. It's available as a nasal spray or injection and is less commonly used due to concerns about its long-term effectiveness and potential side effects.
- **Romosozumab (Evenity)**: This drug is a monoclonal antibody that both increases bone formation and decreases bone resorption. It's used as an injectable treatment for postmenopausal women with a high risk of fracture.
- **Diet and Supplements**:
  - **Calcium**: Essential for maintaining healthy bones. Calcium can be taken as a dietary supplement if dietary intake is inadequate.
  - **Vitamin D**: Helps the body absorb calcium. Supplements are often recommended, especially for those with limited sun exposure or dietary intake.
- **Lifestyle Modifications**:
  - **Exercise**: Weight-bearing exercises like walking, dancing, and strength training can help maintain bone density.
  - **Quit Smoking**: Smoking can decrease bone density.
  - **Limit Alcohol**: Excessive alcohol can lead to bone loss.
  - **Prevent Falls**: Since individuals with osteoporosis have an increased risk of fractures, measures to prevent falls are crucial: Use handrails, wear non-skid shoes, and ensure homes are well-lit. Remove hazards like loose rugs or electrical cords from walking areas. Physical therapy to improve balance may be beneficial.

Paget's Disease

Paget's disease (**osteitis deformans**) is due to a combination of genetic and environmental factors. Some have suggested a viral origin. It is characterized by increased bone breakdown by osteoclasts and compensatory excessive bone formation by osteoblasts. Bones become enlarged, weakened, misshapen, and painful. Bone deformation may occur in the spine, skull, pelvis, femur and tibia. The condition can be confined to one skeletal area or affect multiple bones.

Fractures occur more easily, along with stiff joints, nerve compression, headaches, hearing loss, vision changes, and bowing of long bones.

The diagnosis of Paget's disease is made by imaging (X-ray, CT scan, and radioactive bone scans that show increased bone activity). Serum alkaline phosphatase, a marker of active bone remodeling and turnover, is typically elevated in Paget's; liver function tests can show if the increased alkaline phosphatase originates in the bone or the liver. Biopsy, done on occasion, can provide further confirmation. Blood calcium and phosphorus levels may be normal.

Treatment for Paget's Disease may include bisphosphonates, such as *alendronate, risedronate,* or *zoledronic acid,* to help reduce bone turnover and pain; *calcitonin* to reduce bone resorption and pain. Pain management may include NSAIDs, physical therapy, or corrective surgery, with follow-up monitoring.

Figure 4-6 lists the main causes of hypercalcemia and hypocalcemia.

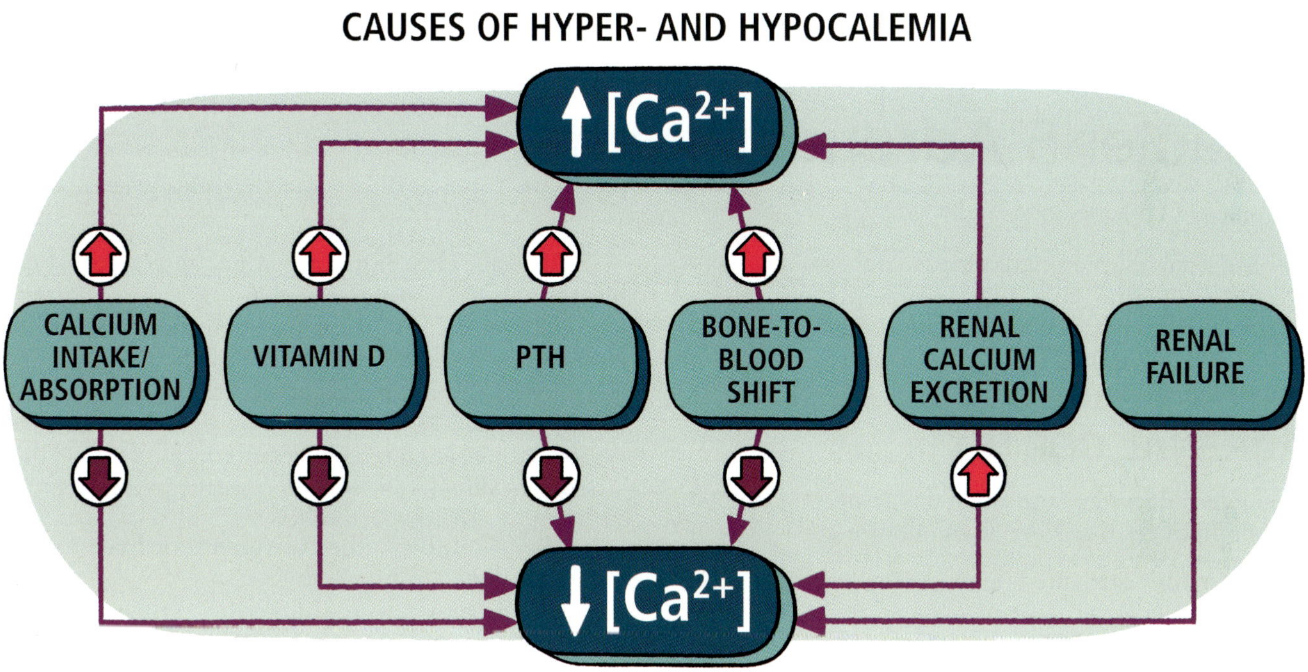

Fig. 4-6. Hyper- and hypocalcemia.

Chapter 5 **Adrenal Glands**

The adrenal (suprarenal) glands are two triangle-shaped endocrine glands that sit atop the kidneys. Each gland has two main zones: the adrenal cortex and the adrenal medulla (**Figs. 5-1** and **5-2**).

ADRENAL CORTEX

The **adrenal cortex**, the outer layer of the adrenal gland, produces three key types of hormone:

1. **Mineralocorticoids** (mainly **aldosterone**) - from the outer (*zona glomerulosa*) layer of the cortex
2. **Glucocorticoids** (mainly **cortisol**) – from the middle (*zona fasciculata*) layer of the cortex
3. **Androgens**, mainly **dehydroepiandrosterone (DHEA)** and **DHEA-sulfate (DHEA-S) -** from the inner (zona reticularis) layer of the cortex (**Figs. 5-1** and **5-2**)

Mineralocorticoids (Aldosterone)

Aldosterone acts on the kidneys to help regulate electrolyte balance by promoting the reabsorption of sodium and excretion of potassium. Sodium reabsorption creates an osmotic effect in which water is passively reabsorbed along with the sodium. This increases blood volume and, hence, blood pressure, while helping maintain electrolyte balance. Aldosterone also helps decrease blood acidity (increase pH) by increasing the kidney secretion of hydrogen ions into the urine and reabsorbing bicarbonate.

Although ACTH has some stimulatory effect on aldosterone secretion, the main stimulus to aldosterone secretion is the renin-angiotensin-aldosterone system (**Figs. 5-2** and **5-3**).

The renin-angiotensin-aldosterone system that stimulates aldosterone secretion works as follows:

- Renin catalyzes the conversion of liver Angiotensinogen to Angiotensin I.
- Lung Angiotensin Converting Enzyme (ACE) catalyzes the conversion of Angiotensin I to Angiotensin II.
- Angiotension II is a vasoconstrictor that also stimulates the adrenal cortex to secrete Aldosterone.

Glucocorticoids (Cortisol)

Often called the *"stress hormone,"* cortisol plays a critical role in the body's response to stress, including physical injury, illness, and psychological stressors. The body responds to stress by releasing cortisol to meet the challenge. Cortisol's functions include:

- *Metabolism Regulation*: Cortisol helps to regulate metabolism by affecting the way the body uses and stores carbohydrates, fats, and proteins. It can increase glucose production for energy.

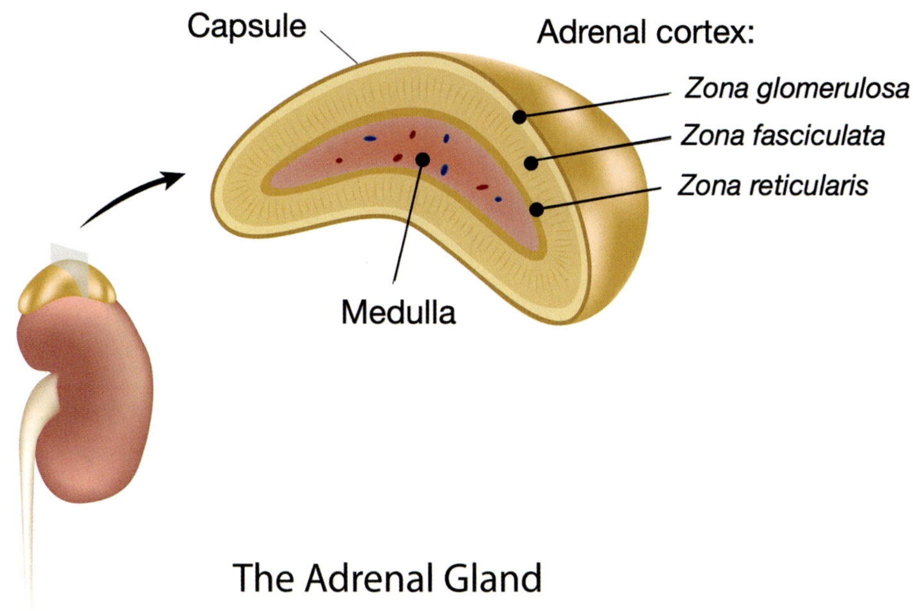

Fig. 5-1. Layers of the adrenal gland.

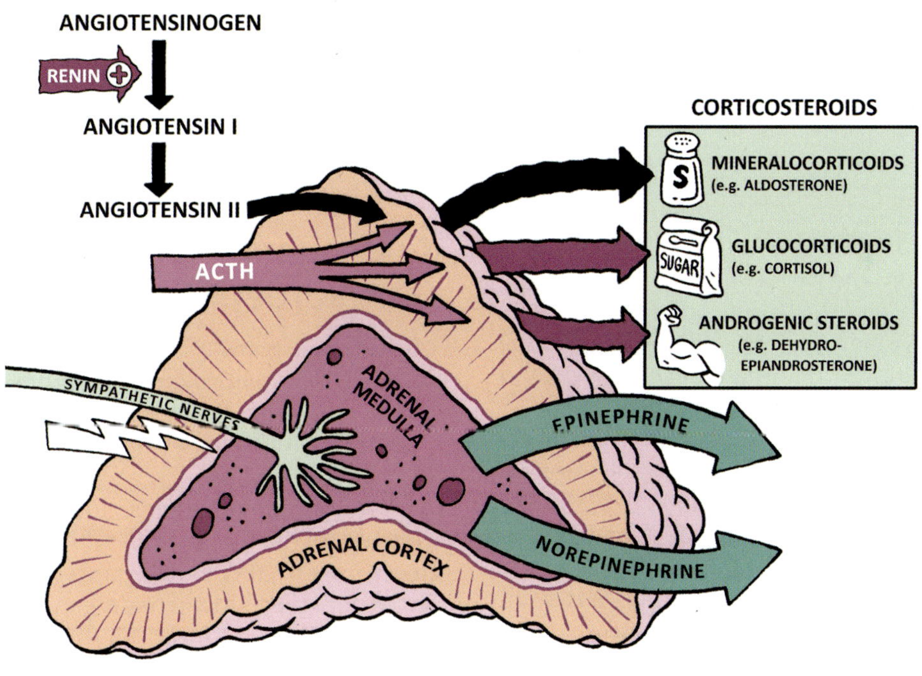

Fig. 5-2. The stimuli to adrenal gland secretion. (From Goldberg, S. Clinical Physiology Made Ridiculously Simple. Medmaster.)

- *Immune System Regulation*: Cortisol has anti-inflammatory properties that can prevent the immune system from becoming overreactive during inflammatory reactions.
- *Blood Pressure Regulation:* Cortisol helps increase and maintain blood pressure by increasing the sensitivity of blood vessel receptors to other hormones that cause the blood vessels to constrict, and by having aldosterone-like effects in promoting sodium and water retention, which help maintain blood pressure and blood volume.
- *Circadian Rhythm*: Cortisol levels naturally fluctuate throughout the day, peaking in the early morning and declining throughout the day and evening.

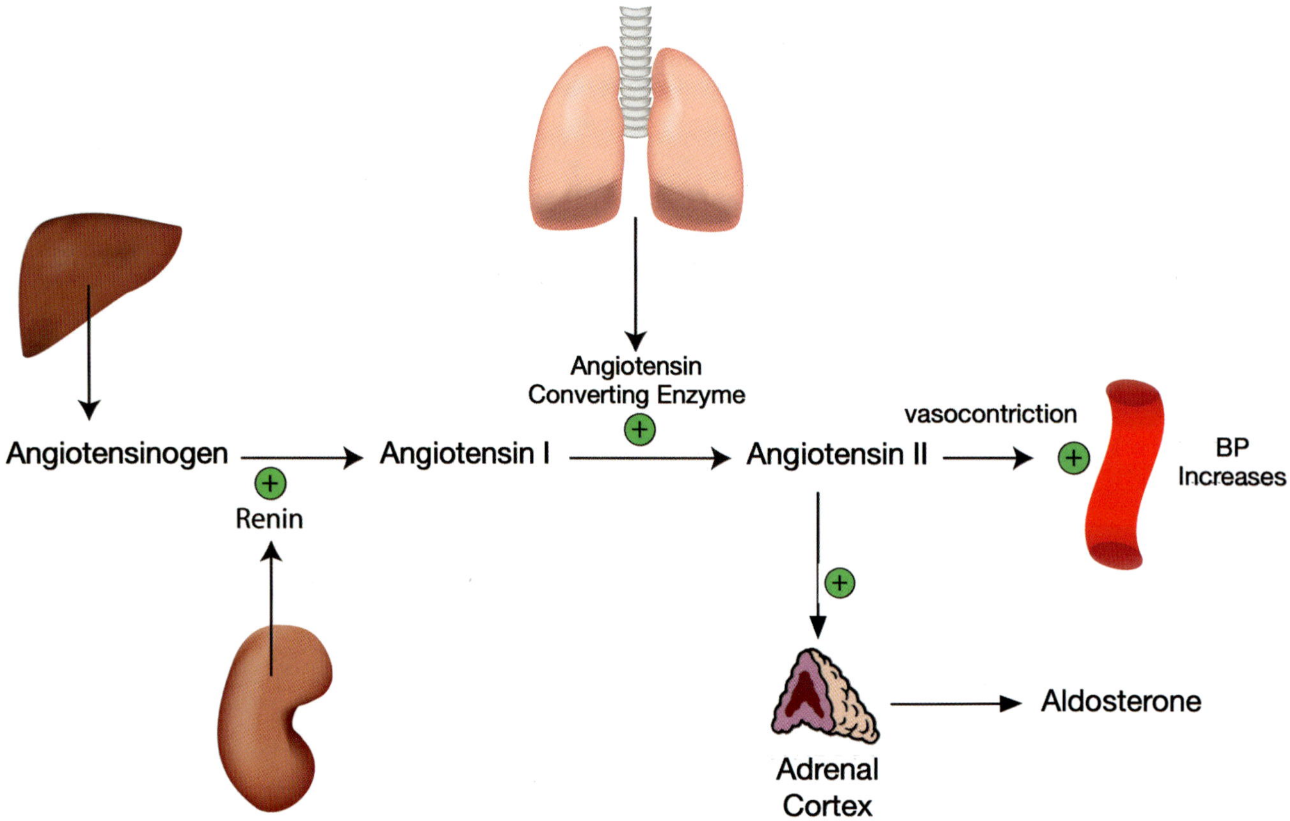

Fig. 5-3. The renin-angiotensin-aldosterone system.

This allows for adequate sleep at night and helps promote energy and alertness in the morning.

- *Development of the Fetus:* In late pregnancy, cortisol plays an important role in the development of the fetus, including the maturation of the lungs and brain.
- *Psychological Effects:* Cortisol, in acute stress situations, can sharpen mental focus and improve cognitive function. Chronic cortisol elevation, though, can have an opposite effect, and lead to mood disorders like anxiety and depression.
- *Bone:* Cortisol may have a positive effect on increasing calcium release from bone to meet immediate physiological needs. However, cortisol can adversely affect bone health by inhibiting intestinal calcium absorption, stimulating osteoclast activity (which leads to bone breakdown) and inhibiting osteoblast activity (preventing bone formation). Chronic elevated cortisol levels may contribute to osteoporosis.

The adrenal glands produce cortisol in response to *ACTH* from the pituitary gland, which in turn is stimulated by *corticotropin-releasing hormone (CRH)* from the hypothalamus (**Fig. 5-4**).

Androgens (Dehydroepiandrosterone; DHEA)

The adrenal gland produces small amounts of male sex hormones (androgens) - **dehydroepiandrosterone (DHEA)**, **DHEA-S** and **androstenedione**. These are precursor hormones that are converted in the peripheral tissues, such as the liver, adipose tissue, and reproductive organs, to testosterone (mainly) and estrogens, e.g., estriol, which are involved in the development and maintenance of secondary sexual characteristics. Most estrogen and testosterone, however, are produced in the ovaries and testes respectively. Also, the ovaries do produce some testosterone, and the testes do produce some estrogen.

- In males, DHEA is mainly converted into testosterone by the enzyme 17 beta-hydroxysteroid dehydrogenase. In females, DHEA can be converted into testosterone and then estrogen through a series of enzymatic conversions involving *aromatase* (aromatization is the enzymatic conversion of androgens into estrogens) (**Fig. 5-9**).

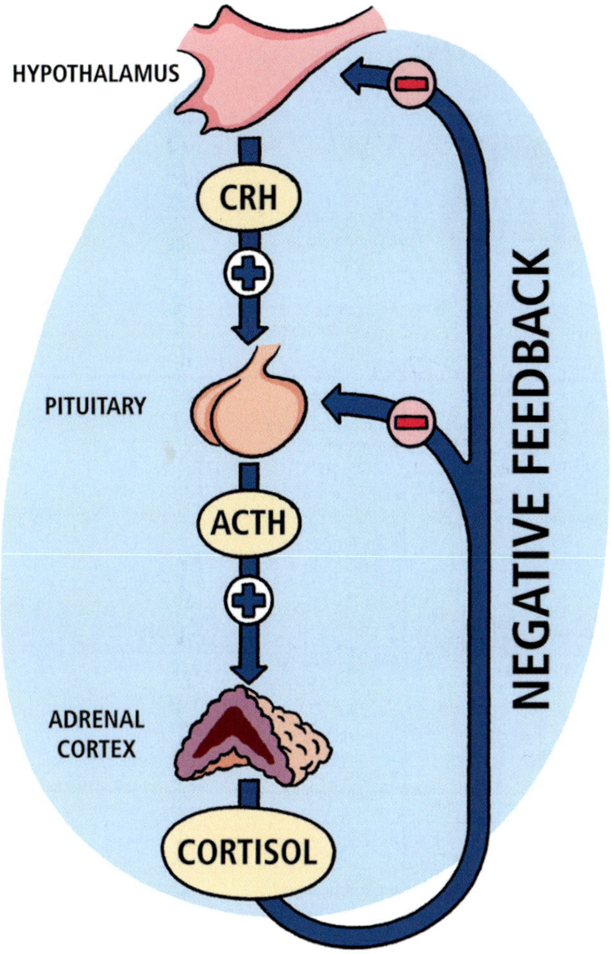

Fig. 5-4. Cortisol feedback to the pituitary gland and hypothalamus. CRH, Corticotropin-Releasing Hormone; ACTH, Adrenal Corticotropic Hormone.

- Testosterone binds to testosterone receptors, and estrogen binds to estrogen receptors located throughout the body, where these hormones do their magic.
- Upon binding to their respective receptors, testosterone and estrogen influence various cellular processes, including those related to sexual development, bone metabolism (promoting bone growth and maintaining bone density) and other functions.

In this book, cortisol, aldosterone, and DHEA are all simply referred to as corticosteroids since they are all steroids and produced in the adrenal cortex. However, when healthcare professionals talk about prescribing corticosteroids, or simply "steroids" as a therapeutic treatment, they usually mean glucocorticoids like prednisone, prednisolone, dexamethasone, hydrocortisone and methylprednisolone. In sports, the term "steroids" is generally used to depict androgenic steroids, which mimic the anabolic muscle-building effects of testosterone.

Cushing's Syndrome

Disorders of the adrenal cortex, such as **Addison's disease** (deficient adrenal cortical hormones) and **Cushing's syndrome** (excess cortisol) can significantly affect body function and require medical management.

Cushing's syndrome (**Fig. 5-5**) can be caused by an adrenal tumor that produces excess cortisol, exogenous administration of glucocorticoid medication, a pituitary adenoma that secretes ACTH (which stimulates the adrenal gland to secrete excess cortisol), an ectopic ACTH-secreting tumor, or a tumor that produces corticotropin-releasing hormone (CRH), which stimulates ACTH production. When the cause is specifically a pituitary tumor that secretes ACTH, that is called **Cushing's *Disease*,** named after Dr. Harvey Cushing, the American neurosurgeon who first described it in 1932.

Figure 5-6 describes the signs and symptoms of Cushing's Syndrome

Causes of Cushing's Syndrome

Causes of cortisol excess (Cushing's syndrome) include:

- *Iatrogenic Cushing's syndrome* from administration of corticosteroids (the most common cause)
- *Pituitary Cushing's syndrome* (*Cushing's Disease*) from overproduction of ACTH by a pituitary tumor
- Ectopic ACTH production (from an ectopic tumor, e.g., in the lungs, pancreas, or thymus)
- *Adrenal Cushing's syndrome* (overproduction of cortisol by a cortisol-secreting adrenal adenoma, carcinoma, or hyperplasia)
- *Multiple Endocrine Neoplasia Type 1* (*MEN1*), *MEN2* and *McCune-Albright syndrome* (fibrous dysplasia of bone, cafe-au-lait spots, and endocrine abnormalities) can predispose individuals to develop Cushing's syndrome.
- In the *Carney complex*, a rare autosomal dominant disorder, there may be cardiac myxomas, excess skin freckling, *overactivity of the adrenal glands*, Schwannomas, breast myxomatosis, and tumors of the testes, thyroid, pancreas or other organs.
- Cortisol resistance, a rare familial condition, causes an increase in ACTH secretion, which causes increased cortisol production to try to compensate for a perceived lack of cortisol. The typical symptoms of Cushing's syndrome do not appear, though, because the body is resistant to cortisol.

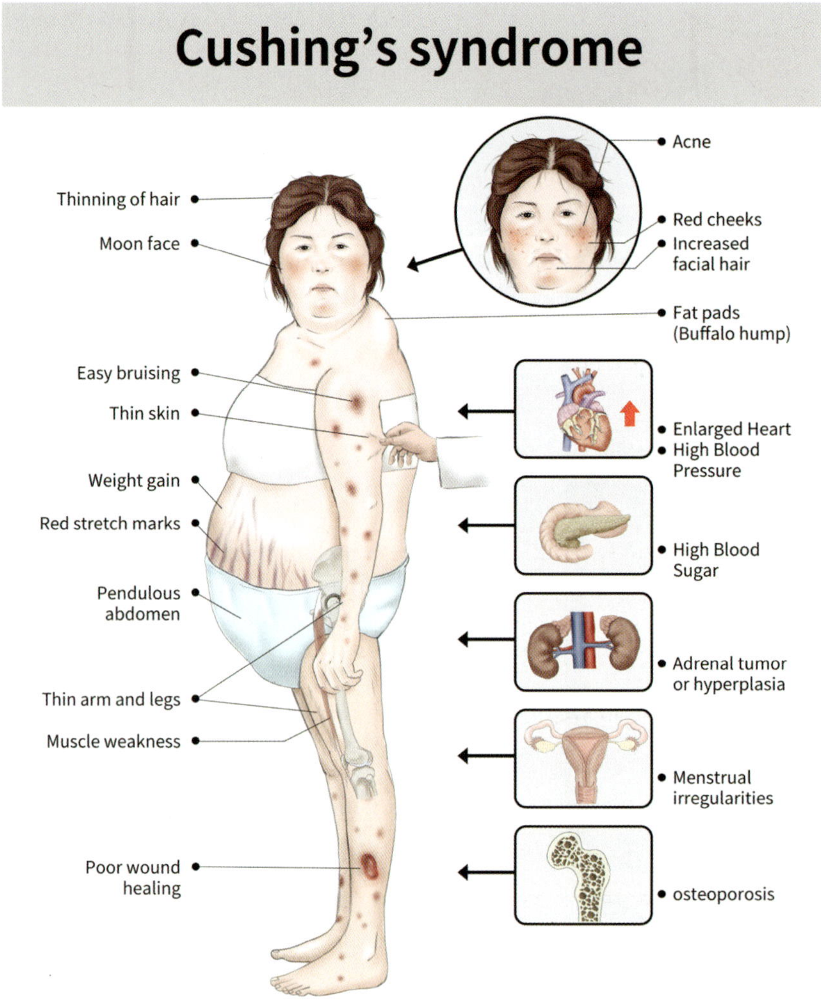

Fig. 5-5. Cushing's syndrome.

Diagnosis of Cushing's Syndrome

The diagnosis of Cushing's syndrome is made through:

- Medical history and physical exam
- Blood tests to measure cortisol, ACTH and other adrenal and pituitary hormones that may be affected in Cushing's syndrome. A cortisol-secreting adrenal tumor can be distinguished from an ACTH-secreting pituitary tumor by noting that the cortisol-secreting adrenal tumor, by negative feedback to the pituitary, results in a *low* ACTH level. ACTH level will be *high*, though, in an ACTH-secreting pituitary tumor that causes excess cortisol secretion (**Fig. 5-4**).
- 24-Hour Urinary Free Cortisol Test: This test measures the amount of cortisol excreted in a 24-hour urine sample. Elevated levels may indicate Cushing's syndrome.
- Salivary cortisol testing (normally shows daily fluctuation, with cortisol levels higher in the morning than in the evening). Cushing's syndrome may show persistently elevated salivary cortisol levels.
- Inferior petrosal sinus sampling of ACTH helps determine if the excess ACTH is coming from the pituitary gland.
- Imaging studies (X-ray, CT, MRI) can visualize the adrenal and pituitary gland size and shape to look for signs of an ACTH-secreting tumor.
- Dexamethasone suppression test (see below)
- CRH (corticotropin-releasing hormone) stimulation test (see below)

Suppression and Stimulation Tests for Cushing's Syndrome

The aim of the suppression and stimulation tests for Cushing's syndrome is to identify the cause of an excess secretion of cortisol. Is it a primarily oversecreting adrenal gland, a pituitary tumor that oversecretes ACTH, or an ectopic ACTH-secreting tumor?

FIGURE 5-6. SIGNS AND SYMPTOMS OF CUSHING'S SYNDROME (CORTISOL EXCESS)
• **Obesity:** Cortisol promotes fat deposition in the abdomen, but lipolysis in the extremities (*central obesity*). It increases appetite and induces insulin resistance, resulting in higher insulin, which causes more fat storage.
• **Amenorrhea:** Cortisol, through negative feedback on the hypothalamus and pituitary gland suppresses not only the production of ACTH but also pituitary luteinizing hormone (LH) and follicle-stimulating hormone (FSH) by inhibiting secretion of gonadotropin-releasing hormone (GnRH) from the hypothalamus. This interferes with the menstrual cycle.
• **Diabetes:** Cortisol, in causing insulin resistance, increases gluconeogenesis to compensate by producing more glucose.
• **Buffalo hump** and **moon face:** Fat accumulates at the base of the neck and in the face. The increased cortisol promotes fat storage and inhibits fat breakdown. The fat storage is typically *central*, away from the arms and legs.
• **Hirsutism:** When ACTH stimulates the adrenal gland to produce excess cortisol, it can also stimulate the secretion of excess adrenal androgens, e.g., DHEA, and androstenedione, which can convert to testosterone in peripheral tissues. In addition, elevated cortisol can induce insulin resistance, which can lead to increased androgen production.
• **Osteoporosis:** Excess cortisol can interfere with the activation of vitamin D, reduce calcium absorption in the intestines, increase excretion of calcium in the kidneys, stimulate osteoclast (bone breakdown) activity and suppress osteoblast (bone building) activity. This decreases bone mass.
• **Stria:** High levels of cortisol can lead to breakdown of collagen in the skin, leading to stretch marks (*stria*).
• **Polycythemia:** Excess cortisol can stimulate the production of erythropoietin and increase the sensitivity of bone marrow to erythropoietin, leading to overproduction of red blood cells.
• **Hypertension:** As part of the stress response, excess cortisol can lead to increased sympathetic nervous system activity, including vasoconstriction. It can also enhance the activity of aldosterone, promoting sodium and water retention in the kidneys, causing increased blood volume and hypertension.
• **Stress ulcers:** Cortisol can divert blood flow from the gastric mucosa as part of the "fight or flight" stress response, and it suppresses immune function, reducing the ability of the mucosal lining to heal and fend off infection.
• **Myopathy:** Muscle protein breaks down for gluconeogenesis.
• **Psychosis:** Cortisol can affect the balance of neurotransmitters in the brain.
• **Decreased inflammatory response:** Cortisol depresses the immune system.
• **Hypokalemic alkalosis:** Excess cortisol can increase the activity of aldosterone, which increases the excretion of potassium in the kidney and reabsorption of sodium ions in exchange for hydrogen ions in the cortical collecting tubule, leaving the blood hypokalemic from decreased potassium, and alkalotic from decreased hydrogen ions.
• **Fatigue:** Sleep disruption, muscle breakdown, impact on mood, and constant readiness for stress wears the body down.

Dexamethasome suppression test: Dexamethasone, a synthetic glucocorticoid, normally suppresses ACTH secretion, and hence cortisol production. (Dexamethasone is the preferred glucocorticoid for this test because it does not interfere with the measurement of cortisol.)

- A normal response to **low dose** dexamethasone is decreased cortisol blood levels, and essentially rules out Cushing's disease. *Why?* In patients with Cushing's disease, which is due to a pituitary ACTH-producing tumor, suppression of cortisone production does not occur with a low dose of dexamethasone because of the autonomous production of ACTH by the pituitary tumor, which resists reacting to dexamethasone. If normal cortisol suppression does occur, this rules out Cushing's disease.
- If normal suppression of ACTH production *doesn't* occur in the *low dose* test, you suspect a poorly-responding ACTH-secreting tumor, but you still have to determine where the ACTH-secreting tumor is, whether in the pituitary gland or ectopic. This can be resolved with a *high-dose* dexamethasone suppression test. The idea is that a pituitary tumor will be suppressed with the higher dose, but an ectopic ACTH-secreting tumor (e.g., a lung cancer) has a mind of its own and still won't suppress, even with a high dose of dexamethasone. This can help distinguish an ACTH-secreting pituitary tumor from the ectopic ACTH-secreting tumor. However, responses among patients may not be so clear-cut, so other confirmatory tests are still needed.

The **CRH (corticotropin-releasing hormone) stimulation test** is another test used to determine whether increased ACTH secretion is due to a pituitary tumor or to an ectopic one. Normally, ACTH secretion *increases* on administering CRH. It will also increase if the problem is with an ACTH-secreting pituitary tumor, but it is less likely to increase with ectopic

ACTH-secreting tumors, which are unresponsive to CRH.

If it is the adrenal gland that is oversecreting the cortisol, this should be elucidated by measuring the ACTH level, which usually will be low in an oversecreting adrenal gland tumor, which suppresses pituitary ACTH secretion. ACTH secretion, though, is typically elevated in an ACTH-secreting tumor, whether it is in the pituitary gland or ectopic.

Treatment of Cushing's Syndrome

Treatment for the cortisol excess in Cushing's syndrome may include:

- Surgery (or in some cases, irradiation) for a cortisol-excreting adrenal tumor (adrenalectomy) or for a pituitary or ectopic ACTH-secreting tumor.
- Medications:
  - *Ketoconazole, metyrapone,* and *mitotane* block enzymes used for cortisol synthesis.
  - *Pasireotide* binds to somatostatin receptors on the pituitary adenoma cells, inhibiting the excess secretion of ACTH from the tumor and hence lowering the levels of cortisol.
  - *Mifepristone* blocks receptors in the tissues that respond to cortisol, thereby inhibiting cortisol's effect.
- Gradual tapering of exogenous corticosteroids is needed to allow the body's natural production of cortisol to resume properly. Rapid withdrawal could otherwise cause withdrawal symptoms of adrenal insufficiency or flare-ups of the disease for which the steroids were originally given.
- Management of accompanying symptoms (e.g., high blood pressure, diabetes, osteoporosis)

Addison's Disease (Primary Adrenal Insufficiency)

Addison's Disease is a disorder of the adrenal cortex that arises from an *undersecretion* of cortisol, aldosterone and adrenal cortical androgens. Different symptoms result from the deficiency of cortisol, aldosterone, or sex hormones:

- *Symptoms from cortisol deficiency:*
  - Fatigue and weakness (decreased cortisol energy metabolism)
  - Gastrointestinal symptoms, e.g., nausea, vomiting, abdominal pain, diarrhea (from increased inflammation and stress from cortisol deficiency)
  - Weight loss and decreased appetite (alterations in metabolism and GI disturbances from deficient cortisol)
  - Hypoglycemia (decreased gluconeogenesis because of decreased cortisol)
  - Mood changes, depression (cortisol influences the central nervous system and the stress response)
- *Symptoms from low aldosterone levels:*
  - Hyponatremia, hyperkalemia, and dehydration
  - Low blood pressure from decreased aldosterone and decreased cortisol. Both normally increase blood pressure.
- *Symptoms from cortical sex hormone deficiency:*
  - Decreased libido, fatigue and weakness, depression and mood swings
  - Menstrual irregularities
  - Reduced muscle mass in men
- *Hyperpigmentation* occurs in Addison's disease due to increased production of melanocyte-stimulating hormone (MSH). This is caused by elevated levels of adrenocorticotropic hormone (ACTH), which shares a common precursor with MSH.

Primary adrenal insufficiency (Addison's disease) can be caused by:

- Autoimmune adrenalitis, which has a genetic predisposition
- Infections (e.g., tuberculosis, HIV / AIDS, or other fungal or bacterial infections)
- Hemochromatosis. (Iron can infiltrate and damage the adrenal gland.)
- Amyloidosis and sarcoidosis. Amyloidosis can cause accumulation of amyloid, while sarcoidosis can form granulomas in the adrenal gland.
- A congenital problem, e.g., congenital adrenal hyperplasia; adrenal dysgenesis
- Bilateral adrenal hemorrhage. (*Waterhouse-Friderichsen syndrome,* from meningococcal infection results in high fever, headache, weakness, rapid breathing, low blood pressure, shock, disseminated intravascular coagulation, and a petechial or purpuric skin rash.)
- Metastatic cancer. However, adrenal insufficiency does not happen with unilateral adrenal metastasis.
- Bilateral removal of the adrenal glands
- Medications. E.g., *ketoconazole* and *etomidate* can interfere with adrenal hormone production.
- Radiation therapy

In **secondary adrenal insufficiency**, the pituitary gland doesn't secrete enough ACTH. *This does not affect aldosterone secretion*, which is mainly controlled by the renin-angiotensin-aldosterone system (**Figs. 5-2** and **5-7**). As a result, while cortisol deficiency may be present, hyponatremia, hyperkalemia, and dehydration are less common, since aldosterone is not compromised. There may still be the other

PRIMARY AND SECONDARY ADRENAL INSUFFICIENCY

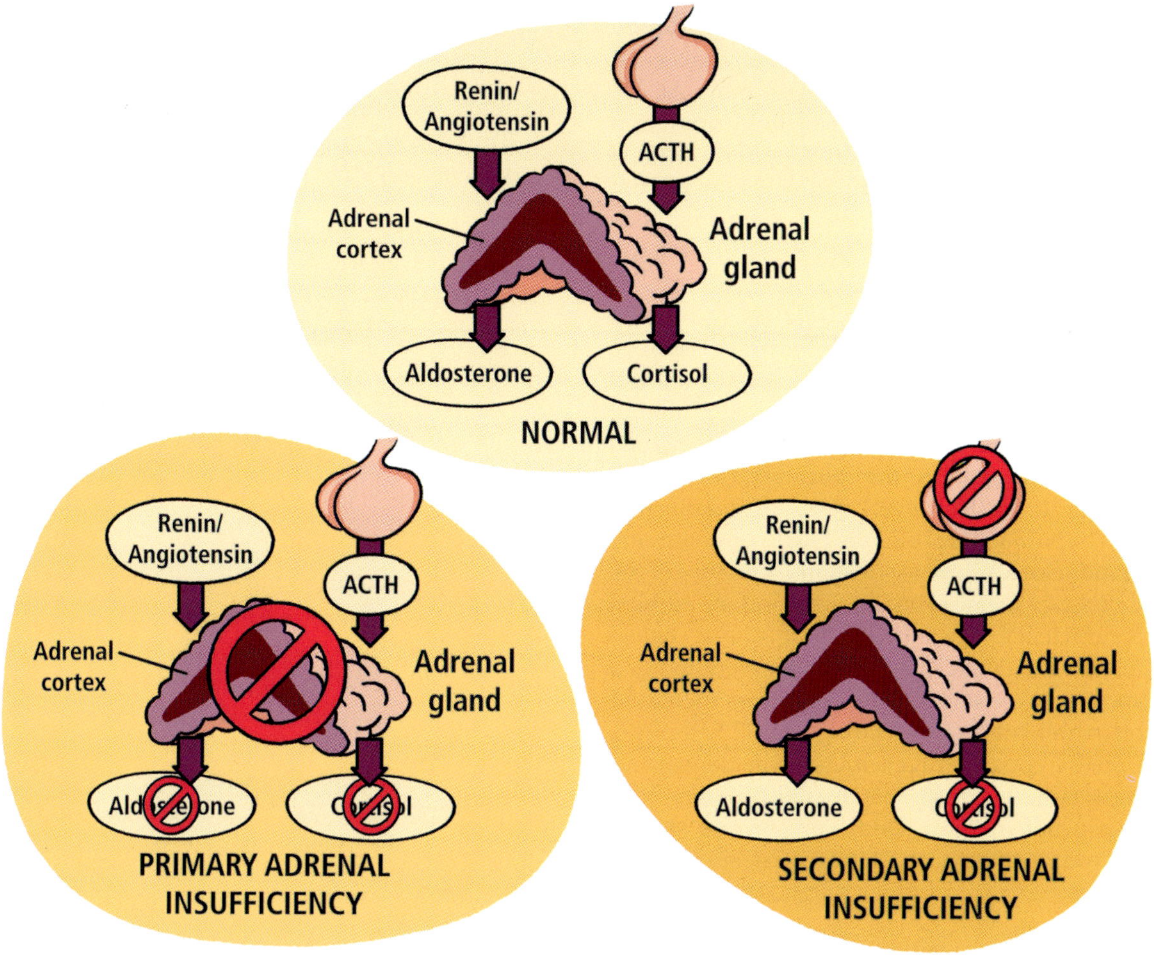

Fig. 5-7. Adrenal insufficiency. (Modified from Berkowitz, A. Clinical Pathophysiology Made Ridiculously Simple. Medmaster.)

signs of Addison's disease, including hypotension. Hypotension, with dizziness and fainting, may arise with cortisol deficiency alone, because cortisol normally plays a role in increasing blood pressure by increasing the blood vessel sensitivity to hormones that cause the blood vessels to constrict (epinephrine and norepinephrine) in the stress of a "fight or flight response." Nor is there the hyperpigmentation found in primary adrenal insufficiency, where ACTH secretion is excessive.

A large pituitary or hypothalamic tumor that causes secondary adrenal insufficiency may cause other pituitary hormone deficits, as well as visual field defects from compression of the pituitary gland and optic chiasm.

The main cause of secondary adrenocortical insufficiency is the administration of exogenous glucocorticoids that are withdrawn abruptly. The symptoms and signs can be severe: *adrenal crisis*, with weakness, vomiting, abdominal pain, low blood pressure, confusion, and hypoglycemia, since the body doesn't have enough time to start producing its own cortisol, which was suppressed by the exogenous steroids.

Diagnosis of Cortisol Deficiency

The diagnosis of cortisol deficiency, apart from considering the symptoms and signs, includes:

- Blood tests:
  - Morning blood or saliva cortisol level. If low, this should prompt further tests for the cause of cortisol deficiency.
  - The ACTH blood level is elevated in primary adrenal insufficiency due to lack of negative feedback to the pituitary; ACTH is low in secondary adrenal insufficiency due to a secretory deficiency originating in the hypothalamus or pituitary gland.

- The **ACTH stimulation test** measures cortisol levels in response to synthetic ACTH (*Synacthen*) injection – cortisol levels remain low in primary adrenal insufficiency (where the adrenals can't function), rather than in acute pituitary ACTH deficiency, where the adrenals do function and can respond to ACTH. In long-term ACTH deficiency, though, the adrenals may not respond to Synacthen, since the adrenal glands may have atrophied or become functionally impaired.
- In the **Insulin Tolerance Test (ITT)**, insulin is administered intravenously to induce hypoglycemia, a stressor that normally should trigger the release of cortisol by stimulating the hypothalamus to release CRH, which in turn stimulates the pituitary to release ACTH. If cortisol levels rise, it suggests that the hypothalamic/pituitary axis and adrenal glands can respond to stress and the cause of the deficiency is not primary or secondary adrenal insufficiency. There may, for instance, be an intermittent deficiency in cortisol secretion or a sub-par secretion that is nonetheless increased on administering of insulin. The ITT, though, causes hypoglycemia, which can be dangerous, especially in elderly patients and others with significant medical conditions. Its use should be weighed against its potential side effects and availability of other diagnostic tests, e.g., stimulation with ACTH.
- Imaging (CT or MRI) can evaluate the pituitary or adrenal glands.

• Antibody testing may reveal anti-adrenal antibodies.

Hyperaldosteronism

Excess or insufficient aldosterone production can result in electrolyte abnormalities, abnormal blood pressure, and fluid imbalances. The problem can originate within the adrenal gland or in the renin-angiotensin-aldosterone system (RAAS). Defects in the pituitary gland do not significantly affect aldosterone secretion, since it is the RAAS, rather than ACTH, that primarily controls aldosterone production. ACTH primarily controls cortisol and DHEA secretion, not aldosterone secretion.

Signs and Symptoms of Aldosterone Excess (Hyperaldosteronism)

- Hypertension (from increased sodium reabsorption and fluid retention)
- Hypokalemia. (Potassium is excreted in exchange for sodium reabsorption.)
- Muscle weakness (low potassium)
- Headaches may occur from hypertension.
- Alkalosis. (H+ is excreted in exchange for sodium reabsorption.)

Primary hyperaldosteronism (**Conn's Syndrome**) is caused by a problem within the adrenal gland, usually an aldosterone-producing benign or malignant adenoma, or bilateral adrenal hyperplasia (enlargement and overactivity of both adrenal glands). In those cases, there is an autonomous overproduction of aldosterone that is not dependent on the renin-angiotensin system. It may be familial.

Secondary hyperaldosteronism is caused by factors outside the adrenal gland. The common causes include conditions that reduce blood flow to the kidneys, decrease blood volume, or lower blood pressure, such as congestive heart failure, cirrhosis with ascites, nephrotic syndrome, and renal artery stenosis, which increase kidney renin secretion (**Figs. 5-2, 5-3, 5-8A** and **5-8B**). The increased aldosterone in this scenario is a physiological response to these conditions, driven by activation of the renin-angiotensin system to restore blood volume and blood pressure.

Secondary hyperaldosteronism may also be due to an aldosterone-secreting ovarian carcinoma or to certain medications. Thiazide and loop diuretics, by volume depletion, can trigger a compensatory increase in aldosterone levels to conserve fluid volume. Licorice-containing products can have an aldosterone-like effect.

In **Liddle syndrome** ("pseudoaldosteronism"), there is an increased sensitivity of sodium channels in the kidney, leading to aldosterone-like effects, with consequent low levels of aldosterone and renin.

Diagnosis of Hyperaldosteronism

The diagnosis of hyperaldosteronism is based on:

- The medical history and physical exam (e.g., early-onset hypertension, hypokalemia, muscle weakness)
- Blood tests:
  - *Aldosterone and renin blood levels*: High aldosterone and *low* renin levels occur in primary hyperaldosteronism, since renin secretion is suppressed by negative feedback from high aldosterone. High aldosterone and *high* renin levels occur in secondary hyperaldosteronism of renal origin due to high renin that initiates the rise in aldosterone. A high aldosterone/renin ratio gives greater accuracy in determining that the hyperaldosteronism has its primary cause in the adrenal gland rather than the kidney.
  - *Blood potassium and sodium concentration*: Sodium concentration in hyperaldosteronism

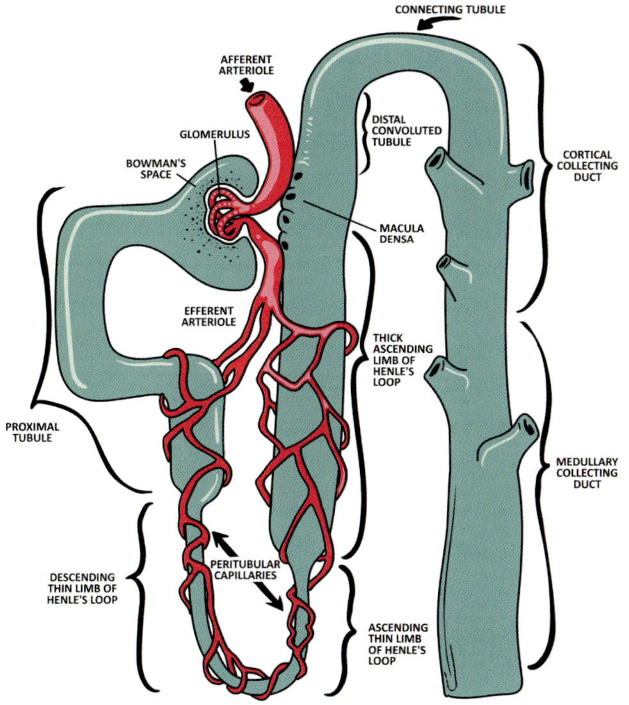

Fig. 5-8A. Overview of the nephron. (From Goldberg, S. Clinical Physiology Made Ridiculously Simple. Medmaster.)

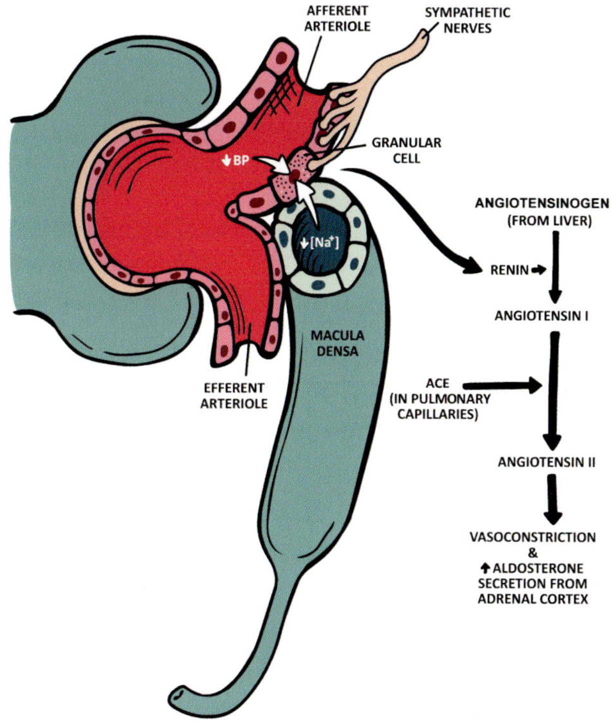

Fig. 5-8B. The juxtoglomerular apparatus. Renin secretion is stimulated by low blood pressure, decreased sodium in the macula densa of the renal tubule, and sympathetic nerve stimulation, resulting in increased aldosterone secretion and increased blood sodium and blood pressure. (From Goldberg, S. Clinical Physiology Made Ridiculously Simple. Medmaster.)

is high, or normal due to other compensatory mechanisms; potassium is low.

- Urinary aldosterone levels (high)
- A 24-hour urine collection for aldosterone levels helps measure aldosterone production and excretion.
- The *saline infusion test* is used to confirm the diagnosis of primary hyperaldosteronism. The increased blood volume from saline infusion normally suppresses aldosterone secretion. In primary hyperaldosteronism, though, the adrenal gland is autonomously secreting aldosterone and is not sensitive to the effects of increased blood volume.
  - *Fludrocortisone suppression test.* Fludrocortisone is a synthetic mineralocorticoid that has similar effects as aldosterone. Normally, aldosterone levels should be suppressed by fludrocortisone, but not in primary hyperaldosteronism, where the adrenal gland autonomously secretes aldosterone.
- Imaging studies. CT, MRI, and kidney ultrasound can visualize the adrenal glands for structural abnormality.
- Adrenal vein sampling. A catheter in an adrenal vein samples aldosterone from each adrenal gland to determine if the problem lies in one or both glands.

Treatment of Hyperaldosteronism

- Mineraldehyde receptor antagonists (e.g., *spironolactone* or *eplerenone*) block the effects of aldosterone.
- Surgery in primary hyperaldosteronism, which may involve an adrenalectomy, can be used to remove an adrenal adenoma or hyperplasia. Unilateral adrenal involvement is usually treated surgically, while bilateral involvement is usually treated medically.
- For secondary hyperaldosteronism, it is important to treat the underlying cause (e.g., renal artery stenosis, heart failure, cirrhosis).
- Diuretics, e.g., thiazides, are used to control blood pressure and reduce fluid retention.
- Decreased dietary sodium intake

Hypoaldosteronism

Primary hypoaldosteronism is the result of conditions that damage the adrenal cortex, leading to decreased aldosterone production. These include Addison's disease (primary adrenal insufficiency) where there is destruction or dysfunction of the entire adrenal cortex, leading to insufficiencies of cortisol, aldosterone, and androgens.

Secondary hypoaldosteronism arises outside the adrenal gland. For instance, it may result from decreased renin from the kidneys.

Signs of hypoaldosteronism include hyponatremia, hyperkalemia, dehydration, and low blood pressure. There may also be a metabolic acidosis, since less sodium is absorbed in exchange for H+ ions.

The causes of hypoaldosteronism include all the causes of adrenal insufficiency that affect the production of cortisol as well, such as Addison's disease and congenital adrenal hyperplasia. Isolated mineralocorticoid deficiency may result from genetic mutations that cause a specific defect in producing aldosterone (e.g., *adrenoleukodystrophy; triple A syndrome; familial hyporeninemic hypoaldosteronism*) or a resistance to aldosterone (e.g., *pseudohypoaldosteronism*).

Advanced renal disease with low renin secretion can be found in some cases of glomerulonephritis, diabetic nephropathy, and polycystic kidney disease, resulting in low aldosterone production. In addition, ACE inhibitors, angiotensin receptor blockers (ARBs), and certain antifungal medications can lead to a reduction in aldosterone secretion.

Diagnosis of Hypoaldosteronism

- Blood tests for levels of aldosterone, renin, sodium and potassium. *Low aldosterone levels with elevated renin coincide with primary hypoaldosteronism. Low aldosterone with low renin coincide with secondary hypoaldosteronism* where the kidney is not producing enough renin. Hyponatremia and hyperkalemia occur with both primary and secondary hypoaldosteronism.
- Adrenal antibody testing may be useful to rule out an autoimmune origin.
- Imaging studies help evaluate the adrenal glands for structural abnormalities or tumor.
- Genetic testing may identify rare genetic disorders that cause aldosterone deficiency.

Treatment of Hypoaldosteronism

The treatment for isolated hypoaldosteronism is hormone replacement (e.g., fludrocortisone, which has mineralocorticoid activity) and salt supplementation where needed. Other hormone supplements may be needed when there is more extensive adrenal insufficiency, as in Addison's disease or congenital adrenal hyperplasia.

Addison's Disease Versus Congenital Adrenal Hyperplasia

Congenital Adrenal Hyperplasia (CAH) is a group of inherited genetic disorders of the adrenal glands, mainly *21-hydroxylase deficiency* (about 95% of cases) and *11-beta hydroxylase deficiency*. These lead to a deficiency in one of the enzymes needed to produce cortisol, and, in some cases, aldosterone (**Fig. 5-9**). The underproduction of these hormones triggers a feedback loop that causes the pituitary gland to release more ACTH. ACTH tries to stimulate the adrenal glands, which enlarge trying to meet the demand for cortisol. The overstimulation of the adrenal glands leads to the overproduction of other hormones not targeted by the genetic mutation, such as the androgen DHEA, which may cause a range of symptoms, including ambiguous genitalia in females, early puberty, and excess body hair.

Addison's disease (primary adrenal insufficiency) involves destruction of the *entire* adrenal cortex, so that *all* the cortical hormones may be deficient, including cortisol, aldosterone, and DHEA. While Addison's disease, like CAH, can be genetic, it can also have other causes, such as infection, metastatic cancer, bilateral adrenalectomy, and hemorrhage.

Addison's and CAH differ in that:

- Addison's symptoms often come on slowly, while the symptoms of CAH can present at birth.
- In CAH, elevated androgen levels can lead to symptoms of virilization in females.

Both CAH and Addison's disease are treated with replacement of the missing hormones, including mimetics of cortisol (hydrocortisone, prednisone, or dexamethasone) and aldosterone (fludrocortisone), as well as increased dietary intake of salt for the hyponatremia of aldosterone deficiency. For CAH, since androgens are commonly overproduced rather than deficient, the cortisol mimetics alone serve to suppress ACTH release and therefore decrease androgen production. Anatomical cosmetic surgery may be considered in females born with ambiguous genitalia due to premature androgen exposure.

Adrenal Crisis

Adrenal crisis is a life-threatening medical emergency, due to a severe deficiency in cortisol. It often occurs in individuals with Addison's disease or other kinds of adrenal insufficiency and can be triggered by stress, severe infection, trauma, or surgery. If untreated, it can lead to shock, organ failure, and death. The treatment

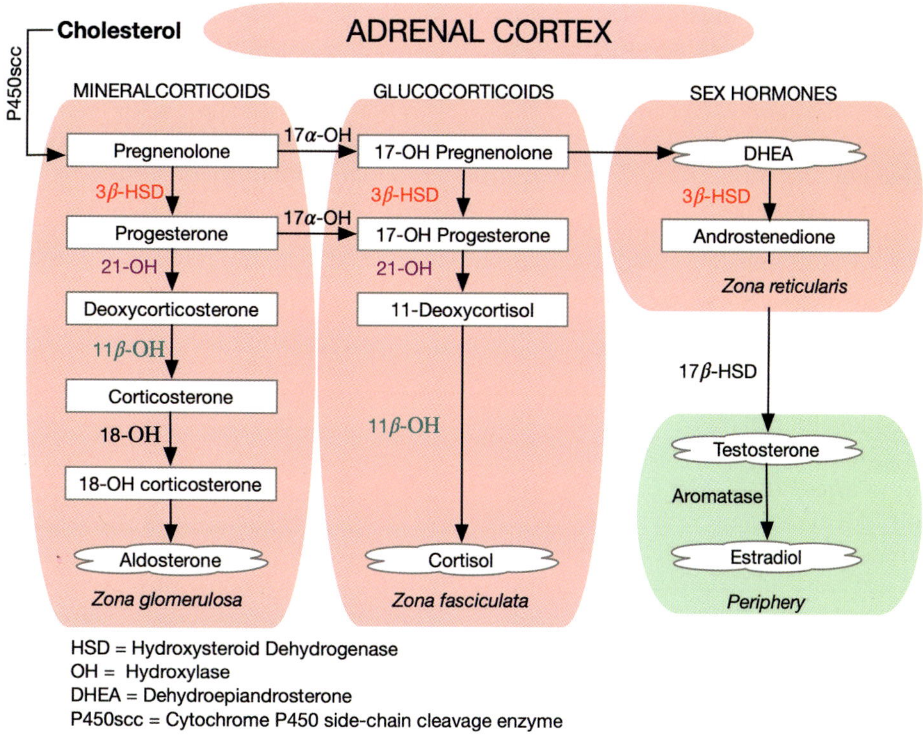

Fig. 5-9. Adrenal hormone synthesis.

includes high-dose intravenous or intramuscular glucocorticoid replacement (e.g., with hydrocortisone) and rehydration with fluids containing sodium, dextrose and water to restore blood pressure and fluid and electrolyte balance, since a deficiency of cortisol and aldosterone can cause hyponatremia, hypoglycemia, and dehydration. Patients with primary adrenal insufficiency may also need fludrocortisone, an aldosterone mimetic, but this may not be necessary if hydrocortisone is used since hydrocortisone itself has some aldosterone-like effects.

DHEA Excess

Dehydroepiandrosterone (DHEA) has androgenic effects; it is converted to testosterone in the periphery. In females, excess DHEA causes masculinization, acne, irregular menstrual cycles, decreased breast size, and mood changes. In males, the effects may be acne, gynecomastia (conversion of testosterone to estrogens), and infertility.

Causes of DHEA Excess

There are a number of ways in which DHEA levels can be excessive:

- Some adrenal tumors can oversecrete DHEA.
- Polycystic ovary syndrome may incur an increase in DHEA.
- In congenital adrenal hyperplasia, deficient cortisol leads to increased ACTH secretion, which stimulates DHEA synthesis.
- In Cushing's disease, increased ACTH production causes increased DHEA production.

Diagnosis of DHEA Excess

The diagnosis of DHEA excess can be made by determining the blood level of DHEA-S, a more stable form of DHEA. A complete hormone panel, including ACTH, cortisol, other adrenal hormones (androstenedione, androstenediol, 17-hydroxyprogesterone), and sex hormone-binding globulin provides a more comprehensive evaluation. Imaging studies such as CT and MRI can help determine whether the cause lies with an adrenal tumor or polycystic ovary. It is also important to note whether the patient is taking DHEA supplements marketed as anti-aging, as DHEA levels naturally decrease with age.

Treatment of DHEA Excess

The treatment of DHEA excess tries to address the underlying condition that causes it (e.g., adrenal gland disorder, polycystic ovary syndrome). Medications may be used that block androgen production (oral contraceptives with *estrogen* and *progestin*) or block androgen receptors (*spironolactone, cyproterone*).

DHEA Deficiency

DHEA deficiency may be marked by fatigue, decreased libido, mood and cognitive changes, weight gain, dry skin and hair, and weakened immune function. It may be caused by Addison's disease, aging, and certain chronic inflammatory conditions.

The diagnosis of DHEA deficiency is facilitated by blood tests assessing levels of DHEA-S, as well as other hormones that might implicate the adrenal glands, pituitary gland, or ovaries/testes. The *Cosyntropin test* may help evaluate DHEA deficiency: Synthetic ACTH is administered to see if it stimulates the adrenal gland to produce DHEA and cortisol. A failure to respond is an indication of adrenal insufficiency.

ADRENAL MEDULLA

The **adrenal medulla**, the inner region of the adrenal gland, produces two main hormones: epinephrine and norepinephrine, both derivatives of the amino acid tyrosine:

Thyroxine←**Tyrosine**→Dopamine→
Norepinephrine→Epinephrine

Epinephrine and Norepinephrine

- **Epinephrine (adrenaline)**, the main hormone secreted by the adrenal medulla, plays a key role in the body response to stress, often called the *"fight-or-flight"* response. Epinephrine increases heart rate, blood pressure, and energy availability to prepare the body for immediate action. Epinephrine can have vasoconstrictor or vasodilator effects. It acts as a vasoconstrictor when acting on *alpha-adrenergic receptors* in blood vessels of the skin, mucous membranes, digestive tract, and kidney, to increase blood pressure and redirect blood flow to essential organs, like the heart, brain, and skeletal muscles during stress. It also acts as a vasodilator, acting on *beta-2 adrenergic receptors* in blood vessels of skeletal muscles and the coronary arteries to increase needed blood flow to the muscles and heart during stress.

  As part of the "fight or flight" response, epinephrine also stimulates the conversion of glycogen in the liver to glucose for added energy, as well as dilation of bronchioles for added oxygen.
- **Norepinephrine (noradrenaline)** works synergistically with epinephrine. However, while epinephrine acts mainly as a hormone, norepinephrine, which is secreted in smaller amounts by the adrenal medulla, acts mainly as a neurotransmitter (in which case the norepinephrine is produced within the secreting neuron rather than the adrenal medulla). Norepinephrine regulates local vasoconstriction and blood pressure within the peripheral nervous system by acting on alpha-1 receptors in arterioles and veins. It also increases heart rate and contractility by acting on beta-1 receptors in the heart muscle. Norepinephrine, as a neurotransmitter in the central nervous system, is also involved in attention, focus, arousal, and the sleep-wake system.

The adrenal medulla is stimulated to release epinephrine and norepinephrine by sympathetic nerves (**Fig. 5-2**), but the neurotransmitter of those incoming nerves is acetylcholine, not norepinephrine.

The use of the nervous system rather than the blood circulation for stimulating the adrenal medulla makes sense, since you want a very fast response for "fight-or-flight" and the nervous system is quicker than the bloodstream route in releasing epinephrine and norepinephrine.

Excess Epinephrine and Norepinephrine

High levels of epinephrine and norepinephrine can cause:

- High blood pressure and rapid heart rate
- Anxiety
- Sweating
- Tremors and muscle twitching
- Dilated pupils (part of the fight-or-flight reaction, letting more light into the eye in threatening situations)
- Increased alertness
- Digestive issues (nausea, abdominal discomfort, diarrhea) from redistribution of blood flow to more vital organs.

Excess epinephrine and norepinephrine can be caused by a catecholamine-secreting tumor, such as pheochromocytoma, paraganglioma, neuroblastoma, or Multiple Endocrine Neoplasia Type 2 (MEN2).

While **pheochromocytoma** usually arises from chromaffin cells in the adrenal gland, it rarely may originate outside along the sympathetic nervous system pathways (**paragangliomas**) in the abdomen, chest, and pelvis. It is marked by episodes of high blood pressure, tachycardia, palpitations, and anxiety. The patient should avoid things that may trigger an attack:

- Excess physical activity
- Stress
- Sudden changes in body position
- Tyramine-rich foods, which can cause a sudden release of stored norepinephrine from nerve endings (e.g., aged cheeses, fermented foods, certain beers, cured meats, overripe fruits, soy products)
- Certain medications:
  - *Sympathomimetics* (e.g., pseudoephedrine found in over-the-counter medication for colds and allergies)
  - Monoamine oxidase inhibitors (MAOI): *MAOI antidepressants*, like phenelzine and tranylcypromine, prevent the normal breakdown of catecholamines. Tricyclic anti-depressants can also increase sensitivity to catecholamines.
  - Anesthetics: Certain anesthetic agents used during surgery (e.g., *ketamine*, *succinylcholine*, epinephrine-containing local anesthetics, *halothane* and histamine-releasing drugs like *atracurium* and *mivacurium*) can provoke symptoms.
  - Contrast dyes in radiology
  - Beta-blockers (unopposed alpha receptor stimulation)
  - Caffeine
  - Corticosteroids (can indirectly enhance catecholamine action)
  - Phosphodiesterase inhibitors (e.g., *sildenafil*, *tadalafil*)
  - Certain antipsychotic medications
  - Glucagon: Used in diagnostic testing and sometimes to treat hypoglycemia; glucagon may provoke symptoms in individuals with pheochromocytoma.
  - Alcohol: Though not a medication, alcohol consumption can provoke an attack in some people.

Diagnosis of Epinephrine/Norepinephrine Excess

Apart from the history and physical exam (increased blood pressure, rapid heart rate, anxiety, sweating), epinephrine/norepinephrine excess can be detected in several ways:

- Blood and urine tests, measuring for excess levels of epinephrine, norepinephrine and their metabolites (metanephrines, vanillylmandelic acid [VMA])
- *CT or MRI scans* can be used to locate a secreting tumor. More than 95% of pheochromocytomas are intra-abdominal.
- *MIBG scintigraphy*. MIBG is a molecule that structurally resembles norepinephrine and is taken up by catecholamine-secreting cells. Radiolabeled MIBG scintigraphy is used to localize tumor "hot spots" that have taken up the MIBG.
- *Clonidine suppression test*. Clonidine normally suppresses the release of catecholamines. If catecholamine levels remain elevated it may indicate pheochromocytoma, which is unresponsive to clonidine.
- *Genetic testing*, e.g., for Multiple Endocrine Neoplasia Type 2 (MEN2) or von Hippel-Lindau syndrome (which manifests as multiple benign and malignant tumors and cysts in different parts of the body and can include pheochromocytomas or paragangliomas)

Treatment of Epinephrine/Norepinephrine Excess

The main treatment for catecholamine-secreting tumors is surgical removal. Radiation or chemotherapy can be used where surgery is not feasible. Alpha-adrenergic receptor blockers (e.g., *phenoxybenzamine*), or calcium channel blockers (e.g., *nifedipine*) can help control blood pressure, typically before surgery. *Metyrosine*, which inhibits the enzyme tyrosine hydroxylase and reduces catecholamine synthesis, can also be used, generally before surgery. Beta-blockers (e.g., *propranolol*) should not be used unless preceded by an alpha-blocker; otherwise, if the beta-blocker is used alone, this may leave unopposed alpha-adrenergic stimulation, which could cause a hypertensive crisis.

A *deficiency* in epinephrine and norepinephrine may result from surgical removal of the adrenal glands or a genetic deficiency in the ability to produce these hormones. It is treated with hormone replacement using synthetic forms of epinephrine/norepinephrine (e.g., *phenylephrine*), as well as glucocorticoids and mineralocorticoids if the adrenal glands as a whole are not working.

Incidentalomas

One of the problems with broad scanning of the body is the increased likelihood of picking up a false positive, leading to unnecessary tests that would not otherwise be done. Yet such findings cannot simply be overlooked. An **incidentaloma** is a coincidentally discovered mass during medical imaging that was not suspected. It is a term commonly used in the context of adrenal incidentalomas, which are adrenal gland tumors discovered incidentally when imaging is performed for unrelated reasons, such as abdominal CT or MRI scans. Adrenal incidentalomas are found in up to 5% of individuals who undergo abdominal imaging.

Incidentalomas can be benign or malignant and may involve various organs or structures, including the adrenal glands, thyroid gland, pituitary gland, kidneys, liver, and other areas. Most of them are benign and do not cause any symptoms or hormonal abnormalities. However, some can be functioning tumors that produce excess hormones, such as cortisol (causing Cushing's syndrome) or catecholamines (causing symptoms of pheochromocytoma).

Diagnosis of Incidentaloma

1. *Medical history and physical examination*
2. *Imaging studies*: The imaging techniques, whether CT scan, MRI, or ultrasound can provide detailed information about the size, location, and characteristics of the mass. Additional imaging studies may be performed to get a better understanding of the mass and its potential impact on surrounding structures.
3. *Laboratory tests*: For an adrenal incidentaloma, hormonal evaluations, such as cortisol, aldosterone, DHEA-S, catecholamine, metanephrine, testosterone, estrogen, renin, and ACTH levels, may be conducted to assess its functional status.
4. *Biopsy or fine-needle aspiration* may be performed to obtain a tissue sample to determine whether the mass is benign or malignant. Biopsy should be done only after a pheochromocytoma has been ruled out by biochemical tests, to avoid a sudden hypertensive crisis precipitated by the biopsy. Pheochromocytomas should undergo surgical resection.
5. *Genetic testing* may be done in particular situations.

Treatment of Incidentaloma

The **treatment** of an incidentaloma depends on its location, size, characteristics, and hormonal activity:

- **Observation and Monitoring**: When the incidentaloma is small, stable in size, and shows no signs of malignancy or functional hormone production, a conservative approach of regular observation and monitoring may do, with periodic imaging studies, blood tests, or other evaluations to assess any changes in the mass over time.
- **Medication**: Medication may be prescribed to manage the hormonal imbalances in a functional adrenal incidentaloma. For example, medications can be used to control excessive cortisol production or block the effects of excess catecholamines. *Ketoconazole*, *metyrapone*, *mitotane*, *etomidate*, and *pasireotide* can inhibit cortisol production. Alpha- and beta-blockers can be used to manage symptoms of excess catecholamines. *Metyrosine* decreases catecholamine synthesis.
- **Surgical Removal**: In certain situations, surgical removal of the incidentaloma may be recommended. This is particularly true for those that are large, growing, causing symptoms, or showing signs of malignancy. Surgical removal may involve minimally invasive techniques, such as laparoscopy or robotic-assisted surgery, or open surgery depending on the specific circumstances and the location of the mass.

Chapter 6 Hypertension

Hypertension (high blood pressure) is a common but potentially serious condition that can lead to significant health complications, including stroke, heart disease, and kidney failure if not properly managed. Treatment for hypertension typically involves lifestyle changes, medications, or a combination of both, and is often tailored to individual patient needs.

What Controls Blood Pressure?

Maintaining an appropriate blood pressure is vital for proper perfusion of tissues and organs. The genius of the body provides several systems that work in concert to regulate blood pressure:

- **Cardiac Output** is the volume of blood pumped by the heart per minute. It's determined by heart rate (the number of heart beats per minute) and stroke volume (the volume of blood pumped out with each beat). Increased cardiac output typically leads to increased blood pressure.
- **Peripheral Resistance** is the resistance of the arterial system, primarily the arterioles. Vasoconstriction increases resistance, leading to increased blood pressure. Conversely, vasodilation decreases resistance, leading to decreased blood pressure.
- **Blood Volume** can influence blood pressure. An increase in blood volume usually raises blood pressure, and a decrease in volume will do the opposite. Blood volume is managed in large part by the kidneys, which regulate fluid balance through urine production.
- The **sympathetic nervous system** can cause vasoconstriction and increase cardiac rate and contractility. Activation of the sympathetic system, as in response to stress or danger, typically raises blood pressure.
- **Baroreceptors**, located in the carotid artery sinuses and in the aortic arch, sense changes in blood pressure. They then signal the brain, which adjusts the blood pressure by altering cardiac output, heart rate, and peripheral resistance (**Fig. 6-1**).
- **Endothelial Factors** in the endothelial wall of blood vessels produce *nitric oxide* (NO), which causes vasodilation and lowers blood pressure in response to hypoxia and other factors, while *endothelin* causes vasoconstriction and raises blood pressure in response to angiotensin II and vasopressin. Both NO and endothelin are paracrine signaling molecules.
- **Blood Viscosity**. The thickness or stickiness of blood can influence pressure. Higher viscosity due to factors like increased red blood cell count can increase resistance and blood pressure.
- **Elasticity of Arteries**: Healthy, elastic arteries can expand and contract with each heartbeat, helping to moderate blood pressure. With atherosclerosis, arteries become stiffer, leading to increased blood pressure.

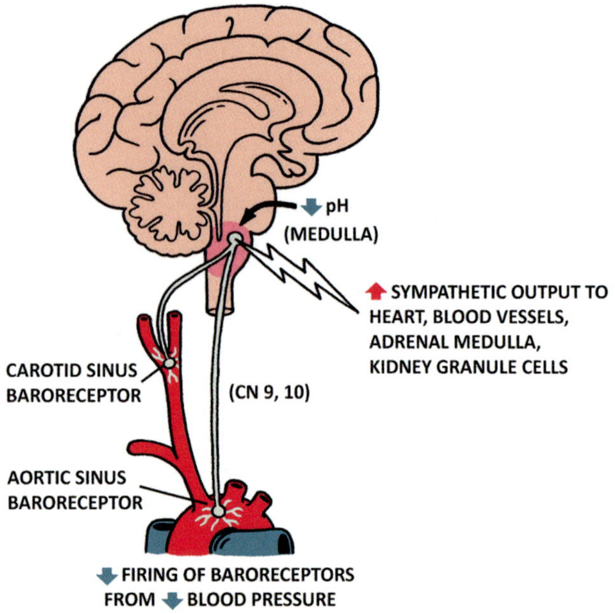

Fig. 6-1. Decreased blood pressure detected by baroreceptors in the aortic and carotid sinuses, as well as decreased pH, signal the brain stem to increase sympathetic output and raise blood pressure. CN, Cranial Nerve. (From Goldberg, S. Clinical Physiology Made Ridiculously Simple. Medmaster.)

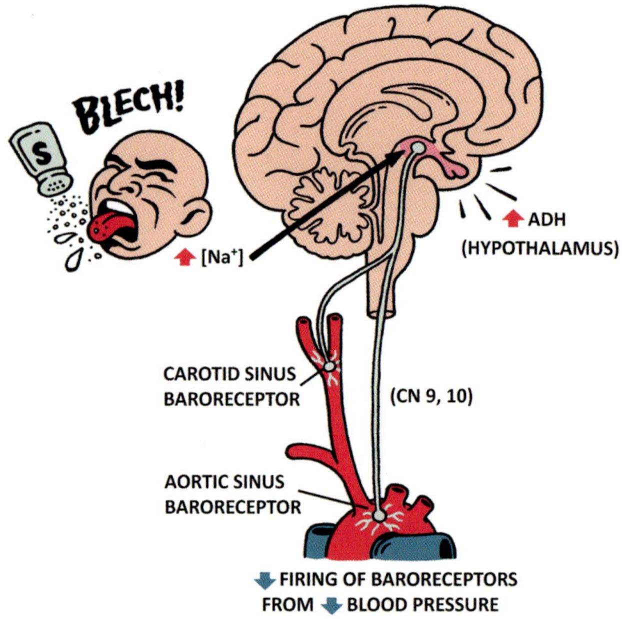

Fig. 6-2. Increased serum osmolality, particular from sodium, stimulates ADH secretion in the hypothalamus, resulting in increased fluid retention and increased blood pressure. CN, Cranial Nerve. (From Goldberg, S. Clinical Physiology Made Ridiculously Simple. Medmaster.)

- **Hormones**: Various hormones influence blood pressure:
  - **Epinephrine and Norepinephrine** raise blood pressure by increasing heart rate and causing vasoconstriction.
  - **Antidiuretic Hormone (ADH; vasopressin)**, released by the posterior pituitary, promotes water retention in the kidneys, increasing blood volume and blood pressure (**Fig. 6-2**). It also has vasoconstrictive effects.
  - **Renin-Angiotensin-Aldosterone System (RAAS)**: Renin is produced by the juxtaglomerular cells of the kidney (**Fig. 5-8A** and **5-8B**). It initiates the renin-angiotensin-aldosterone system, a chemical cascade involved in regulating blood pressure, fluid balance, and electrolyte homeostasis. Renin catalyzes the conversion of angiotensinogen, a protein produced by the liver, into angiotensin I. Angiotensin I is converted into angiotensin II by angiotensin-converting enzyme (ACE), produced largely by the lungs. Angiotensin II is a vasoconstrictor that also stimulates aldosterone release from the adrenal glands, as well as sodium and water reabsorption in the kidney.

Renin release (**Fig. 5-8A** and **5-8B**) is stimulated by:

1. Low blood pressure, as reflected in the afferent arteriole of the kidney
2. Decreased sodium chloride concentration detected by macular densa cells in the thick ascending limb of the loop of Henle
3. Sympathetic nervous system stimulation of the juxtaglomerular cells of the kidney
   - **Atrial Natriuretic Peptide (ANP)** and **B-type Natriuretic Peptide (BNP)**, in counterbalance to epinephrine/norepinephrine, ADH, and the renin-angiotensin-aldosterone system, *lower* rather than raise blood pressure. ANP is released by cardiac atrial muscle, BNP by ventricular muscle in response to stretching from increased blood volume and pressure. These hormones decrease blood pressure by promoting salt and water excretion by the kidneys, and vasodilation. BNP elevation is used as a marker for heart failure.

All these factors work in a complex interplay to ensure that tissues and organs receive adequate blood flow under a wide range of conditions. Disruptions in these systems can lead to hypertension or hypotension.

What Causes High Blood Pressure?

There are two main types of hypertension:

1. **Primary (essential) hypertension**: This is the most common type, affecting most individuals

who have hypertension. The exact causes are not known, but several factors are believed to play a role:

Genetics: Hypertension tends to run in families.

Age: The risk of hypertension increases as people get older, due to arteriosclerosis.

Ethnicity: Some ethnic groups, especially African and Afro-Caribbean populations, have a higher risk of developing hypertension.

Salt Sensitivity: Some people are more sensitive to salt, which can increase blood pressure.

Obesity: Being overweight or obese increases the risk of hypertension. Particularly at risk are individuals who have visceral obesity (fat around the visceral organs, as opposed to subcutaneous fat).

Physical Inactivity: Lack of regular exercise can contribute to weight gain and increases the risk of hypertension.

Diet: High intake of salt and saturated fats, and low intake of potassium can contribute to increased blood pressure.

Alcohol Consumption: Chronic excessive alcohol intake can raise blood pressure.

Tobacco Use: Smoking and chewing tobacco can cause the blood vessels to narrow, leading to increased blood pressure.

Stress: Chronic stress may contribute to hypertension, especially if it leads to poor habits like unhealthy eating or smoking.

2. **Secondary hypertension**: This type results from an underlying condition or medication. Causes include:

Kidney Disease: Issues with the kidneys, especially chronic kidney disease, can cause hypertension. The kidneys become less effective in excreting sodium and water and may secrete more renin.

Hormonal Disorders: Hypersecretion of aldosterone, cortisol, epinephrine/norepinephrine, pituitary growth hormone, thyroid hormone, parathyroid hormone, insulin, renin, or antidiuretic hormone can cause hypertension. Tumors like pheochromocytoma can produce epinephrine and norepinephrine.

Medications: Some medications, including certain pain relievers, cold remedies, birth control pills, some prescription drugs, and excess licorice can raise blood pressure.

Pregnancy: Some women experience hypertension during pregnancy, known as *gestational hypertension* or, when more pronounced, *preeclampsia*. Preeclampsia may be difficult to distinguish symptomatically from pheochromocytoma, as both can have hypertension, headaches, and proteinuria.

Vascular Diseases: Conditions like coarctation of the aorta can cause hypertension.

Drugs: Stimulants, such as cocaine or amphetamines, can raise blood pressure.

Evaluating the Cause of Hypertension

The approach to evaluating the cause of hypertension includes:

Personal History: When was hypertension first diagnosed? Are there any previous readings available? What medications is the patient taking? Some drugs can raise blood pressure, including NSAIDs, oral contraceptives, decongestants, some antidepressants, and others. What is the patient's lifestyle regarding salt and alcohol intake, physical activity, tobacco use, and dietary habits? Are there any symptoms suggesting secondary causes (e.g., sleep apnea, sweating and palpitations from pheochromocytoma, muscle weakness or cramps, suggesting hyperaldosteronism)? **Family history**: Has any immediate family member been diagnosed with hypercholesterolemia, hypertension, or related conditions?

Previous health conditions: Diabetes, high cholesterol, kidney disease, or any other relevant conditions

Physical Examination:

- **Blood pressure measurement**: Measure blood pressure in both arms, and consider measuring in a leg if there is suspicion for coarctation of the aorta (e.g., weak femoral artery pulse in comparison with radial artery pulse).
- **Body mass index (BMI)**: Calculate BMI to assess overweight or obesity. The BMI is calculated by dividing an individual's weight in kilograms by their height in meters squared (or [weight in pounds divided by height in inches squared] x 703). A BMI over 25 is considered overweight; over 30 is obese. High BMI values (typically above 30) are associated with an increased risk of obesity-related health issues.
- **Heart**: Check for murmurs, irregular rhythms, or other abnormalities.
- **Lungs**: Listen for any rales, which might suggest heart failure.
- **Abdomen**: Palpate for enlarged kidneys, masses, or abnormal aortic pulsation.
- **Neck**: Examine for thyroid enlargement or bruits.
- **Eyes**: Check for signs of hypertensive retinopathy, e.g., arteriolar narrowing, hemorrhages and exudates, papilledema.

- **Lower extremities**: Look for edema and check pulses.

Laboratory and Diagnostic Tests:

- **Basic blood tests**: Complete blood count (CBC); basic metabolic panel to evaluate kidney function (creatinine, BUN) and electrolytes.
- **Urinalysis**: Check for protein, blood, or other abnormalities that might suggest kidney disease.
- **Lipid profile**: Assess for dyslipidemia, a cardiovascular risk factor.
- **Electrocardiogram (ECG)**: Look for evidence of left ventricular hypertrophy, arrhythmias, or other cardiac issues.
- **Other tests based on suspicion**: Plasma renin, aldosterone, and cortisol levels, urine catecholamines, and imaging, like renal ultrasound, CT scan, or MRI if a secondary cause of hypertension is suspected

Further Testing for Secondary Hypertension, if there's a clinical suspicion of secondary hypertension based on history, physical exam, or initial tests:

- **Renal artery imaging**: For suspected renal artery stenosis
- **24-hour urine collection**: For aldosterone, cortisol, or catecholamines if considering conditions like hyperaldosteronism, Cushing's syndrome, or pheochromocytoma
- **Sleep study**: If obstructive sleep apnea is suspected, as sleep apnea is a risk factor for hypertension

Evaluation of Cardiovascular Risk: Consider age, gender, smoking status, cholesterol levels, and other factors to assess overall cardiovascular risk.

Treatment of Hypertension

Treatment for hypertension typically involves lifestyle changes, medications, or a combination of both:

Lifestyle Changes:

- **Diet**: The *Dietary Approaches to Stop Hypertension (DASH) diet* is often recommended. The DASH diet focuses on:
  - *High Intake of Fruits and Vegetables*: These provide fiber, vitamins, and minerals like potassium and magnesium, which help control blood pressure.
  - *Whole Grains*, rather than white, refined grains to help control blood sugar
  - *Lean Protein*: Including fish, poultry, and legumes while minimizing red meat and processed meats like sausages and hot dogs
  - *Low-Fat or Non-Fat Dairy*: Provides necessary calcium and protein without the added saturated fat
  - *Nuts and Seeds*: In moderation, these provide healthy fats and other nutrients.
  - *Limited Sodium*: The standard DASH diet advises no more than 2,300 mg of sodium per day, while the lower sodium DASH diet recommends no more than 1,500 mg per day.
  - *Limited Sweets and Added Sugars*: The DASH diet recommends minimizing sugar-sweetened beverages and sweets.

People on the DASH diet can significantly lower their blood pressure within weeks, according to several studies. The diet may offer other health benefits, such as weight loss and diabetes risk reduction.

- **Weight Management** can have a significant impact on lowering blood pressure (see **Chapter 20**).
- **Physical Activity** like walking, jogging, cycling, or swimming for at least 150 minutes per week or 75 minutes per week of vigorous exercise can lower blood pressure.
- **Limit Alcohol and Caffeine Intake**.
- **Quit smoking**, as tobacco use can exacerbate hypertension and increase the risk of heart disease. Nicotine is a vasoconstrictor and stimulates the sympathetic nervous system to release catecholamines. It can also damage the endothelial lining of blood vessels, impairing their ability to dilate.

Medications for High Blood Pressure:

- **Renal-acting:**
  - **Carbonic Anhydrase Inhibitors** (e.g., *acetazolamide*) are weak diuretics (now only rarely used) that reduce the absorption of bicarbonate ions, which are excreted along with sodium, indirectly affecting sodium and water reabsorption.
  - **Loop Diuretics** (e.g., *furosemide*) reduce sodium and potassium reabsorption (**Fig. 6-3**).
  - **Thiazide Diuretics**, such as *hydrochlorothiazide* lower blood pressure by increasing the excretion of sodium and water (**Fig. 6-3**).
  - **Potassium-sparing Diuretics** (e.g., *spironolactone, amiloride*) inhibit aldosterone and decrease sodium reabsorption and potassium excretion (**Fig. 6-3**).
  - **Renin Inhibitors**, such as *aliskiren*, inhibit the enzymatic action of renin, which normally activates the renin-angiotensin-aldosterone pathway.
  - **Vaptans** (**aquaretics**, e.g., *tolvaptan*) inhibit antidiuretic hormone (ADH) receptors in the

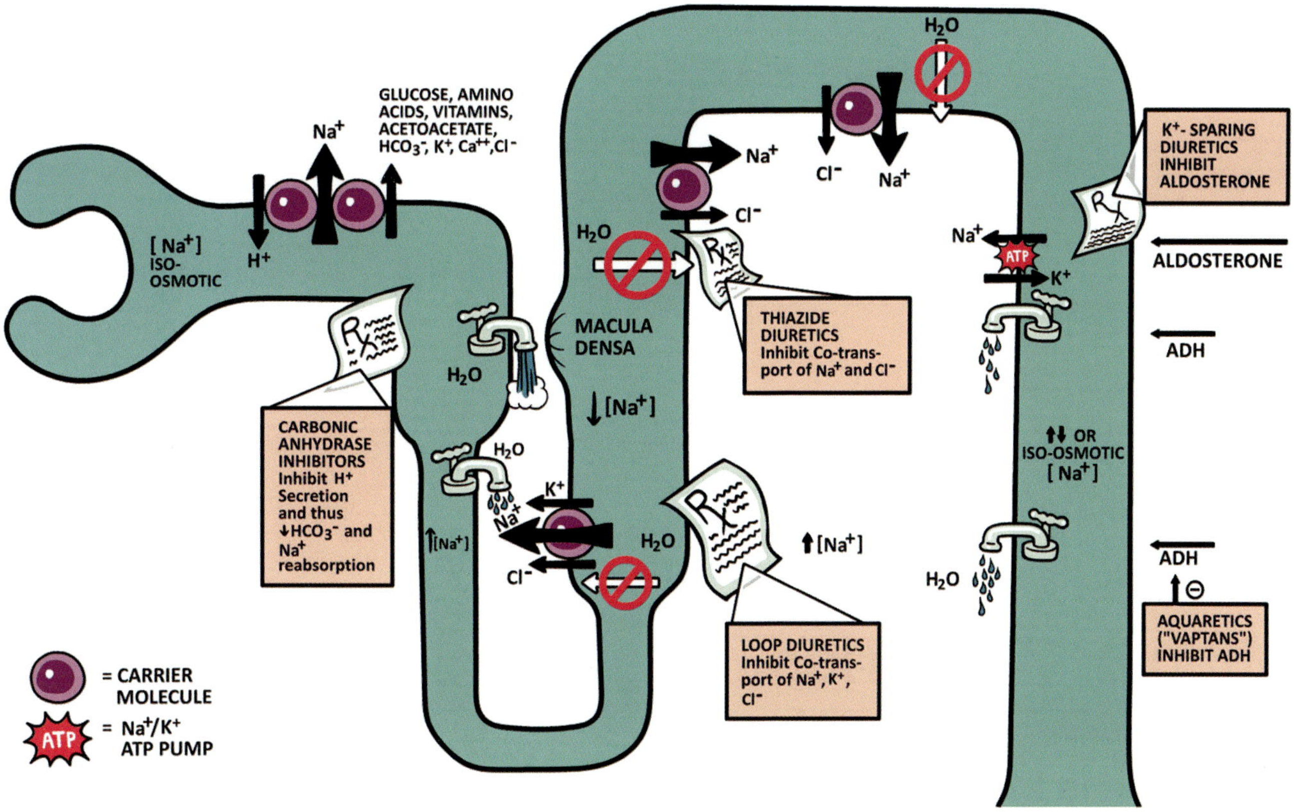

Fig. 6-3. Sites of action of antihypertensive drugs in the renal tubule. (From Goldberg, S. Clinical Physiology Made Ridiculously Simple. Medmaster.)

kidney and hence inhibit water reabsorption. They have only a mild anti-hypertensive effect, though, as they remove water but not sodium, and are more useful in the control of hyponatremia by reducing body water.

- **ACE Inhibitors**, such as *lisinopril* and *enalapril*, block the conversion of angiotensin I to angiotensin II, a vasoconstrictor that also stimulates the secretion of aldosterone.
- **Angiotensin II Receptor Blockers (ARBs)** like *losartan* and *valsartan* block the action of angiotensin II.
- **Angiotensin Receptor Neprilysin Inhibitors (ARNI)**, e.g., *Entresto*, a combination of *valsartan* (an ARB) and *sacubitril*. Sacubitril blocks the breakdown of natriuretic peptide by the enzyme neprilysin, thus decreasing blood pressure by promoting salt and water excretion by the kidneys, as well as vasodilation.
- **Calcium Channel Blockers**, such as *amlodipine* and *nifedipine*, inhibit the movement of calcium into blood vessels, thereby relaxing the blood vessels and reducing vascular resistance.
- **Beta Blockers** like *atenolol* and *metoprolol* block the effects of epinephrine.
- **Alpha Blockers**, such as *doxazosin*, block alpha-1 adrenergic receptors in blood vessels, which leads to vasodilation and a decrease in vascular resistance and blood pressure.
- **Centrally Acting Drugs** like *clonidine* stimulate alpha-2 adrenergic receptors in the central nervous system, which inhibits the release of norepinephrine and subsequently reduces sympathetic nervous system activity, leading to vasodilation and a decrease in heart rate and blood pressure.
- **Vasodilators**, such as *hydralazine*, directly dilate blood vessels and reduce vascular resistance.

Chapter 7 **Ovaries**

Estrogen and Progesterone

The ovaries serve several crucial functions:

- **Oogenesis**. The ovaries produce, store and release ova (eggs). Starting at puberty they release one ovum (ovulation) during each menstrual cycle for possible fertilization by a sperm cell.
- **Hormone production**:
  - **Estrogen** (a term that includes estradiol, estrone, and estriol) is responsible for the development and regulation of the female reproductive system and secondary female sexual characteristics, e.g., breast development and body shape. It also plays a role in cardiovascular function by decreased low-density lipoprotein (LDL; "bad" cholesterol) and increasing high-density lipoprotein (HDL; "good" cholesterol). Estrogen helps maintain bone density as well.

  Estrogen is synthesized in various body tissues, including ovarian follicles, adipose tissue, placenta, testes, adrenal glands, and other peripheral tissues. It is present in small amounts in men, and plays a role in modulating libido, erectile function, and spermatogenesis.
  - **Progesterone**. During the menstrual cycle, after ovulation, the follicle that released the egg changes into a **corpus luteum** (**Fig. 7-1**). The corpus luteum secretes progesterone, which helps prepare the uterine endometrium for pregnancy, as well as prepare the mammary glands for milk production during pregnancy. If fertilization does not occur, progesterone levels drop, leading to menstruation.

  The placenta takes over progesterone secretion after the first trimester of pregnancy. A small amount of progesterone is also produced by the adrenal glands. Progesterone can slightly elevate body temperature, which is often observed after ovulation.
- **Menopause transition**. With aging, the ovaries decrease hormone production, leading to *menopause*, when menstrual cycles stop. This transition can lead to various symptoms like hot flashes, night sweats, and mood changes.

The Menstrual Cycle and Pregnancy

Prior to puberty, which usually occurs between ages 11 and 15 in girls, there are no menstrual cycles, as the production of FSH and LH is insufficient. Both FSH and LH are necessary for the proper preparation of the uterus for pregnancy. FSH stimulates the growth of the ovarian follicles, which produce estrogen and release the ovum. LH triggers follicular ovulation and transformation of the follicle to a corpus luteum, which secretes both estrogen and progesterone.

The sequence of events in the menstrual cycle is as follows (**Fig. 7-1**):

1. The normal menstrual cycle, on the average, occurs about once every 28 days. Day 1 of

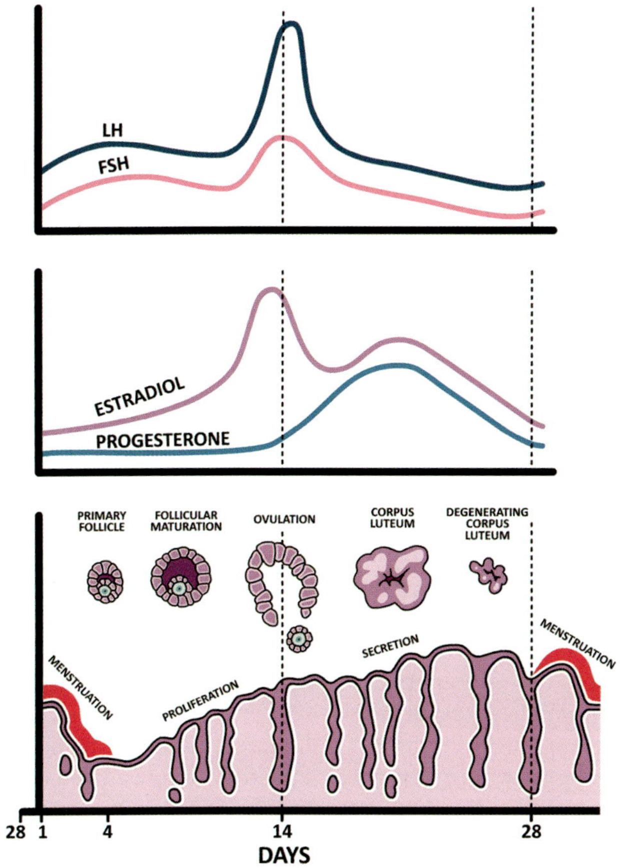

Fig. 7-1. The menstrual cycle. (From Goldberg, S. Clinical Physiology Made Ridiculously Simple. Medmaster.)

the menstrual cycle coincides with the onset of menstruation, which usually lasts about 4-5 days. FSH during this time stimulates the ovarian follicles to mature and produce estrogen, which then induces proliferation of the uterine endometrium. (Actually, a group of follicles enlarges at the beginning of the cycle, but after the fifth or sixth day, a single one of them grows to reach a size of about 2 cm, whereas the others degenerate.) In addition to estrogen secretion, the mature follicle contains the ovum to be fertilized after ovulation. Days 1-13 of the cycle are referred to as the *follicular*, or *proliferative phase* of the cycle.

2. In the usual 28-day menstrual cycle, ovulation occurs about day 14. A menstrual cycle, though, may normally be 21-35 days long. Usually, regardless of the length of the menstrual cycle, ovulation occurs about 14 days prior to menstruation.

   Just prior to ovulation there is an increase in estrogen and, to some degree, progesterone, coinciding with the follicular maturation. The estrogen, in addition to its effects on uterine proliferation, triggers a sudden increase in the pituitary production of LH and FSH, particularly LH. (The direct stimulus to both LH and FSH secretion is hypothalamic gonadotropin-releasing hormone, GnRH. A peculiarity of this arrangement is that GnRH must be released from the hypothalamus in pulses. Continuous administration of GnRH will not stimulate FSH and LH secretion.) The surge in LH secretion induces ovulation, i.e., the release of the ovum, which then begins its trip into the peritoneal cavity, fallopian tubes, and uterus.

3. The increase in LH production stimulates not only ovulation but the development of the corpus luteum, which produces not only estrogen, but significant amounts of progesterone. Progesterone causes the uterus to enter a new phase beyond the proliferative stage, the *luteal phase*, in which there are endometrial secretory gland development and secretion, to prepare the uterine endometrium for implantation of the ovum, should the ovum be fertilized.

4. If fertilization does not occur, the increased estrogen and progesterone from the corpus luteum, and another luteal hormone, *inhibin*, feeds back to the pituitary gland, causing decreased LH and FSH production; the corpus luteum therefore can no longer be maintained and degenerates.

   Estrogen itself appears to have a paradoxical effect on LH and FSH secretion, in that rising levels of estrogen in the early part of the cycle stimulate FSH and LH secretion, whereas chronic presence of estrogen suppresses FSH secretion.

   The estrogen and progesterone in birth control pills suppress ovulation, mainly by inhibiting FSH and LH secretion. The dominant ovarian follicle then can't develop without FSH and there is then no rising estrogen to trigger the LH surge and ovulation. Excess progesterone also thickens the cervical mucus, making it less receptive to sperm. It also decreases fallopian tube motility.

   Chronic excess progesterone also renders the endometrium atrophic, a reason why it is given in large amounts in endometriosis, to control the ectopic pathologic areas of endometrial development. In the "morning-after" pill, a large dose of estrogen and progesterone thickens the endometrium, which then sloughs on withdrawal of the hormones.

   With degeneration of the corpus luteum in the normal menstrual cycle, estrogen and progesterone production decrease; the uterine endometrium can no longer be maintained, and sloughs (menstruation). (Menstrual blood normally does not clot, as the sloughing endometrium releases a fibrinolysin that inhibits clotting.) The decrease in estrogen and progesterone at this time is noted by the hypothalamus (as a decrease in negative estrogen and progesterone feedback), causing a renewal of LH and FSH production, thereby initiating a new menstrual cycle, which begins with growth of new ovarian follicles.

5. If fertilization occurs, it generally happens in the fallopian tube. The ovum can be fertilized within only about a day after ovulation. Since sperm remain viable for only about 1-3 days, intercourse must take place within about a day or so before or after ovulation for fertilization to occur. The trick is to know precisely when ovulation occurs, which is not always a simple matter. One index, although not absolutely reliable, is the rise in basal body temperature, which occurs just after ovulation and persists for the last half of the menstrual cycle.

   The fertilized egg reaches the uterus about 3-4 days after its fertilization in the lateral end of the fallopian tube but does not implant in the endometrium until 3-5 days later.

6. Implantation causes the uterus to quickly produce hCG (human chorionic gonadotrophin), a hormone that has effects similar to LH. This maintains the corpus luteum, ensuring a continuing supply of estrogen and progesterone during pregnancy and preventing the uterine endothelium from sloughing. Actually, the placenta itself is capable of estrogen and progesterone secretion in the last 2 trimesters of pregnancy, so the corpus luteum is not needed in those times. The placenta develops from a fusion of embryonic and maternal issues, along with a closely interdigitating blood supply that connects the maternal and fetal circulations via diffusion to and from the mother and fetus.

   The rapid rise in hCG provides the basis for pregnancy testing. One can detect elevated hCG levels of pregnancy as early as 8 days after ovulation, even before the first missed period. hCG elevation peaks about 2 months into pregnancy, thereafter declining to reach a steady state that lasts from about 6 months to the end of pregnancy.

   The primordial follicles gradually decrease in number through the years, eventually leading to menopause, where their disappearance means a decrease in the production of estrogen and progesterone.

   Clomiphene is a drug that inhibits estrogen feedback receptors in the hypothalamus, thereby increasing the production of GnRH and gonadotrophic hormones. It is used to treat infertility in women with hypothalamic deficiency. Alternatively, infertility can be approached by the administration of measured doses of LH and FSH.

How Do Birth Control Pills Work?

Birth control pills work mainly by suppressing ovulation via negative feedback on the hypothalamic-pituitary-ovarian axis. Most birth control pills contain synthetic forms of estrogen and progesterone (*progestrin*), although some contain only progestrin.

The estrogen and progestrin inhibit the secretion of luteinizing hormone (LH) and follicle-stimulating hormone (FSH) from the anterior pituitary by negative feedback. This prevents the LH surge that is necessary for ovulation, thereby inhibiting the release of an oocyte from the ovarian follicle. Progestrin also thickens the cervical mucus, creating a barrier to sperm and also alters the endometrial lining, making it less receptive to a fertilized ovum.

The "morning after" pill is an emergency measure designed to prevent pregnancy following unprotected intercourse. It will not terminate an existing pregnancy. One type is a progestrin (*levonorgestrel*), which prevents ovulation (and is not considered an abortifacient) and loses effectiveness if ovulation has already taken place. It is most effective if taken within 3 days of unprotected intercourse.

While the levonorgestrel pill and regular birth control pills both act similarly in preventing ovulation, birth control pills are designed to provide a steady level of hormones throughout the menstrual cycle to consistently inhibit ovulation. Levonorgestrel in the morning-after pill, though, is high-dose, for immediate inhibition of the LH surge, to inhibit ovulation as quickly as possible; it is intended for single emergency use.

Another type of "morning-after" pill contains *ulipristal acetate,* which mainly prevents ovulation but possibly also prevents implantation of an already fertilized egg by binding to the progesterone receptor in the endometrium. It is most effective if taken within 5 days of unprotected sex. Whether ulipristal is considered an abortifacient depends on what one considers to be an abortion; is it any time after fertilization of the egg, or only after implantation of the embryo? Hence, the cultural controversy over using ulipristal.

Drugs that terminate an established pregnancy include *mifepristone* (blocks the action of progesterone that is necessary for maintaining the uterine lining), *misoprostol*, *dinoprostone* and *oxytocin* (induce uterine contractions), and *methotrexate* (interferes with DNA synthesis and cell division).

Hyperestrogenism

The symptoms and signs of estrogen excess in women include:

- Irregular menstrual periods
- Breast tenderness and swelling
- Mood swings and irritability
- Water retention. (Estrogen may stimulate the kidney's ability to retain sodium and water.)
- Weight gain (particularly in the abdomen and hip, from water retention plus changes in fat distribution)
- Fatigue, headaches, decreased libido, insomnia
- Digestive issues (nausea or changes in bowel habits)
- Acne
- Increased risk of blood clots
- Increased risk of hormone-dependent cancers, such as breast cancer.

Hyperestrogenism in men can cause gynecomastia, decreased libido, infertility, emotional changes, weight gain, especially around the abdomen and chest, muscle loss, hair loss, fatigue, and possibly an increased risk of prostate cancer.

Hyperestrogenism can be caused by:

- An estrogen-producing tumor (ovarian, testicular, adrenal, benign or malignant)
- Estrogen replacement therapy
- Obesity. Fat tissue contains aromatase enzyme activity, which converts androgens into estrogens.

Diagnosis of Estrogen Excess

Estrogen excess (estrogen dominance) can be diagnosed by:

- The medical history (irregular menstrual periods, breast tenderness, mood swings, weight gain, changes in libido)
- Physical exam (breast changes, excessive body fat distribution)
- Hormone blood levels (increased estradiol, estrone and / or estrone)
- Hormone ratio assessment (increased ratio of estrogen to other hormones, e.g., progesterone or testosterone)
- Estrogen metabolite testing, FSH levels (decreased with excess estrogen), or imaging studies in some cases to assess the ovaries or another possible origin of excess estrogen.

Treatment of Estrogen Excess

Treatment for estrogen excess may include:

- Lifestyle modifications (balanced diet, exercise, stress management)
- Treating the underlying cause
- Aromatase inhibitors, which inhibit the conversion of androgens into estrogens. These include *anastrozole*, *letrozole*, and *exemestane*, although these are usually used to treat estrogen-receptor-positive (ER+) breast cancer. Tamoxifen, another medication used to treat ER+ breast cancer, acts by blocking estrogen receptors on the cancer cells, preventing estrogen from binding, thereby inhibiting tumor growth.

Estrogen Deficiency

The signs of estrogen deficiency include:

- Irregular or absent menstrual periods
- Hot flashes, night sweats. (Estrogen influences the hypothalamus, which helps regulate body temperature by dilation and constriction of blood vessels and sweating.)
- Vaginal dryness
- Urinary symptoms (frequency, urgency, incontinence). Vaginal atrophy can indirectly affect urinary function, contributing to irritation or infection in the urinary tract.
- Mood changes and irritability
- Sleep disturbances
- Decreased libido
- Cognitive changes, memory and concentration difficulty
- Osteoporosis

Estrogen deficiency may be caused by:

- Menopause
- Premature ovarian insufficiency (loss of ovarian function before the age of 40)
- Genetics (e.g., Turner syndrome or Fragile X syndrome)
- Side effects of chemo / radiotherapy
- Anorexia nervosa. (Body fat normally produces estrogen, but if fat is low, disruption of the hypothalamic-pituitary-ovarian axis may occur and may also happen with nutritional deficiency and stress.)
- Surgical removal of the ovaries

Diagnosis of Estrogen Deficiency

- Medical history (hot flashes, vaginal dryness, night sweats, decreased libido, mood changes, changes in menstrual patterns)

- Physical exam (decreased fullness of breast tissue; dry, thin skin; hair thinning; hirsutism sometimes, from a relative increase in androgens)
- Blood levels of estradiol, estrone, estriol, and progesterone (decreased)
- FSH and LH (elevated; more hypothalamic GnRH is secreted due to decreased estrogen feedback.)
- Bone density scan (decreased bone density)

Treatment of Estrogen Deficiency

- Hormone replacement therapy (HRT) (estrogen orally, patches, gels, creams, injectable, or skin implants). There is concern, though, about an increased risk with HRT of developing blood clots and breast or uterine cancer (the risk for uterine cancer can be reduced by adding progesterone). The risks of HRT must be weighed against the risks of remaining estrogen deficient, which include menopausal symptoms, osteoporosis and heart disease.
- Local estrogen for vaginal dryness (vaginal creams, tablets, or rings)
- Lifestyle modification (a balanced diet rich in calcium and vitamin D, exercise, avoiding smoking and excess alcohol)
- Treat underlying conditions (e.g., hypothyroidism or autoimmune conditions if present).
- For menopausal hot flashes, which may involve changes in hypothalamic sensitivity, certain SSRIs (Selective Serotonin Reuptake Inhibitors) and SNRIs (Serotonin-Norepinephrine Reuptake Inhibitors) have been found effective for some, as has *clonidine*, an antihypertensive that acts on brain regions involved in body temperature regulation).

Polycystic Ovary Syndrome (PCOS)

Polycystic ovary syndrome (PCOS) is a hormonal disorder that affects about 5-10% of women of reproductive age. Its main features include:

1. **Irregular Menstrual Cycles**: Women with PCOS often experience irregular or infrequent menstrual periods. This is due to hormonal imbalances that disrupt normal ovulation.
2. **Excess Androgen Levels**: Women with PCOS may have higher levels of androgens, such as testosterone. This can lead to symptoms like acne, hirsutism, and male-pattern hair loss.
3. **Ovarian Cysts**: Multiple small cysts may develop on the ovaries, but not all women with PCOS have cysts. The cysts are immature follicles that have not developed and released an egg during ovulation (**Fig. 7-2**).
4. **Metabolic Disturbances**: PCOS is often associated with insulin resistance, which can lead to elevated blood sugar levels and an increased risk of developing type 2 diabetes. Type 2 diabetics may have high levels of insulin, which can stimulate ovarian androgen synthesis in the theca cells of the ovary. Additionally, women with PCOS may have higher levels of cholesterol and may be at a higher risk of developing cardiovascular diseases.

Other common symptoms and signs associated with PCOS include weight gain or difficulty losing weight, fatigue, mood swings, sleep disturbances, and fertility problems.

Diagnosis of PCOS involves a combination of medical history, physical examination, blood tests to assess hormone levels (including androgens and insulin, which may be elevated) and ultrasound imaging to evaluate the ovaries.

The management of PCOS focuses on symptom control, reducing the risk of complications, and improving overall health. Treatment options may include lifestyle modifications (such as weight loss, exercise, and a healthy diet), hormonal contraceptives (synthetic forms of estrogen and progesterone) to regulate menstrual cycles, medications to manage insulin resistance (e.g., *metformin*) and androgen levels (e.g., *finasteride*, an anti-androgen), and fertility treatments for women trying to conceive (e.g., clomiphene for ovulation induction; in vitro fertilization).

Premenstrual Syndrome (PMS)

Premenstrual syndrome is a complex condition that may present with a variety of symptoms, including

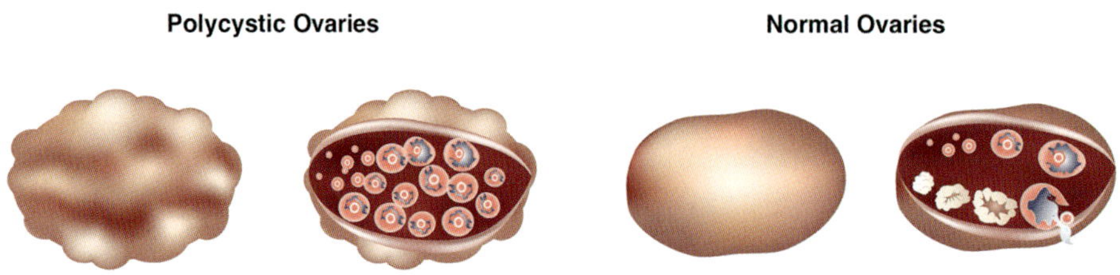

Fig. 7-2. Polycystic ovaries.

mood swings, irritability, breast tenderness, bloating and fluid retention, headache, muscle and joint pain, fatigue, constipation or diarrhea, dizziness, sleep disturbances, food craving for sweet or salty foods, and decreased libido. It typically occurs in the luteal phase of the menstrual cycle, between ovulation and the start of menstruation. PMS likely relates in part to heightened sensitivity to the normal hormonal fluctuations in estrogen and progesterone during the menstrual cycle. Treatment may be multifaceted, involving a balanced diet, exercise, and/or medication, such as NSAIDs for pain, birth control pills for hormonal regulation, and sometimes cognitive behavioral therapy.

Amenorrhea

Amenorrhea is the absence or cessation of menstrual periods in women of reproductive age. The different causes of amenorrhea can be classified into two main categories: **primary amenorrhea** and **secondary amenorrhea (Fig. 7-3).**

Secondary Amenorrhea: Secondary amenorrhea is defined as the absence of menstruation for a period of 3 months or more in women who previously had regular menstrual cycles. Common causes include:

- *Pregnancy*, the most common cause of secondary amenorrhea
- *Hormonal imbalances*: Conditions such as polycystic ovary syndrome, thyroid disorders, hyperprolactinemia (prolactin inhibits the secretion of GnRH from the hypothalamus), or hypothalamic dysfunction can disrupt the hormonal balance necessary for regular menstruation. Pituitary tumors, Sheehan syndrome (postpartum pituitary necrosis) or other pituitary/hypothalamic disorders can create hormonal imbalance. Stress can also disrupt the hypothalamic-pituitary-ovarian axis.
- *Weight-related issues*: Significant weight loss, excessive exercise, or eating disorders like anorexia nervosa can lead to hormonal changes that result in amenorrhea.
- *Structural abnormalities*: Uterine abnormalities, such as fibroids or *Asherman's syndrome* (intrauterine adhesions), can interfere with menstruation.
- *Medications and treatments*: Some medications, such as hormonal contraceptives, certain antipsychotics, antidepressants, and chemotherapy drugs, as well as radiation therapy, can cause amenorrhea. Spironolactone has anti-androgenic properties, but androgens form part of the hormonal balance needed for a regular menstrual cycle. Antihistamines can sometimes raise prolactin levels.
- *Chronic medical conditions*, e.g., chronic kidney disease, liver disease, diabetes mellitus, or certain autoimmune disorders can disrupt hormone balance.
- *Premature ovarian insufficiency*, where there is a premature decline in ovarian function before the age of 40. Natural menopause typically occurs around the age of 45-55.
- *Inflammatory conditions*: Pelvic inflammatory disease (PID) or other chronic inflammatory conditions may affect the reproductive organs.

Primary Amenorrhea: Primary amenorrhea is when a girl has not experienced her first menstrual period by the age of 15 or within 3 years after the start of breast development (*thelarche*). Potential causes of primary amenorrhea include the same ones as secondary amenorrhea, plus a few others:

- *Structural abnormalities*: Malformations or obstructions in the reproductive organs, such as congenital absence of the uterus (*Müllerian agenesis*) or imperforate hymen, can prevent menstruation.
- *Hormonal disorders*: Conditions such as hypothalamic-pituitary dysfunction (e.g., Kallmann syndrome - inadequate GnRH secretion and anosmia), polycystic ovary syndrome (PCOS), or congenital adrenal hyperplasia (CAH) can cause primary amenorrhea.
- *Chromosomal abnormalities*: E.g., individuals with Turner syndrome (45,X) are anatomically female but may lack functional ovaries.
- *Genetic mutation*: The individual may be genetically male (46,XY), but have external female genitalia without a uterus or functional ovaries (e.g., *androgen insensitivity syndrome* (46,XY); *Swyer syndrome*, where the individual develops as female because the cells of the body cannot respond to the male-determining effects of the Y chromosome).

Diagnosis of Amenorrhea

The evaluation of amenorrhea involves a combination of clinical history, physical examination, and various diagnostic studies to determine the underlying cause. The specific tests depend on the clinical history and physical exam findings:

- **Pregnancy Test**: An initial step in evaluating amenorrhea in reproductive-age women is to rule out pregnancy with a urine or serum human chorionic gonadotropin (hCG) test.
- **Blood Tests**:
  - *Hormone Levels*: Assessing levels of thyroid-stimulating hormone (TSH), prolactin, follicle-stimulating hormone (FSH), luteinizing

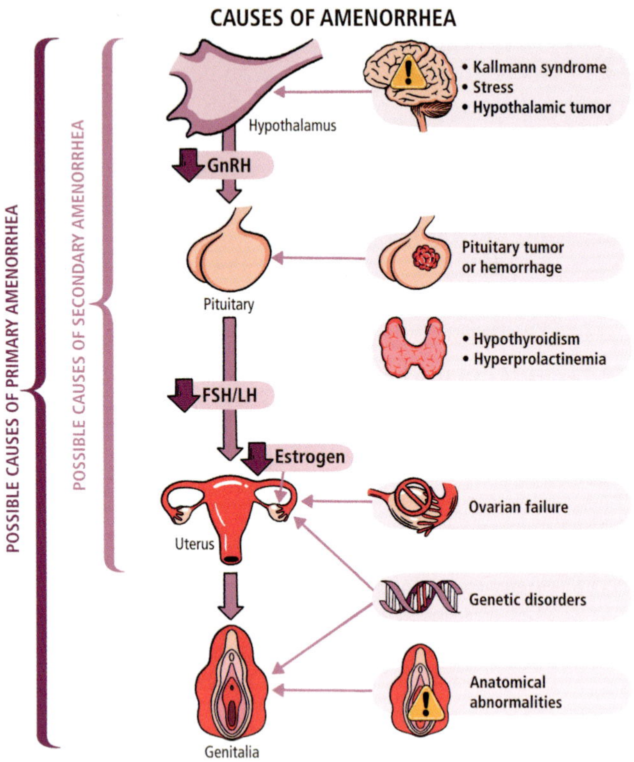

Fig.7-3. Causes of primary and secondary amenorrhea.

hormone (LH), estradiol, progesterone, and androgens (testosterone, DHEA-S) can help identify hormonal imbalances that might be causing amenorrhea.

- *Progestin Withdrawal Test*: Administering progestin (like medroxyprogesterone acetate) can help determine if the amenorrhea is due to a lack of estrogen. If bleeding occurs after withdrawal, it indicates that there is enough estrogen to prime the endometrium, but not enough progesterone decline to cause menstruation, perhaps due to anovulation. If bleeding does not occur, it suggests either that estrogen levels were too low to prime the endometrium or there is an outflow tract obstruction.

- **Imaging Studies**:
  - *Pelvic Ultrasound* helps visualize the uterus, ovaries, and other pelvic structures. It can identify anatomical abnormalities or the presence of ovarian cysts.
  - *MRI* of the brain can assess the appearance of the pituitary gland, especially if there's suspicion of a pituitary tumor causing elevated prolactin levels.
  - *Hysterosalpingography* or *Sonohysterography* are used less commonly but can help evaluate the uterine cavity and fallopian tubes.
- *Karyotyping* studies the individual's chromosomes. It's used if there's suspicion of a chromosomal abnormality, such as Turner syndrome.
- *Endometrial Biopsy*: In certain cases, a small sample of tissue taken from the uterine endometrium can help assess its state and rule out endometrial atrophy or malignancy.
- *Laparoscopy* is not commonly used just for the evaluation of amenorrhea, but it can help identify conditions like endometriosis.

Treatment for Amenorrhea

The treatment for amenorrhea depends on its underlying cause. An appropriate treatment plan can then be followed:

1. **Hormonal Imbalances**:
   - *Polycystic ovary syndrome (PCOS):* Lifestyle changes such as weight loss, regular exercise, and dietary modifications may be recommended. Hormonal medications, such as oral contraceptives or anti-androgens, can help regulate menstrual cycles.
   - *Hypothyroidism*: Treatment includes hormone replacement therapy with synthetic thyroid hormone to restore normal thyroid function. Treatment of hyperthyroidism may also be beneficial.
   - *Hyperprolactinemia*: Dopamine agonists, such as *bromocriptine* or *cabergoline*, are used to lower prolactin levels and restore normal menstrual function.
   - *Premature ovarian insufficiency* or *menopause*: Hormone replacement therapy (HRT) may be prescribed to alleviate symptoms and restore hormonal balance.
2. **Weight-Related Issues**: If amenorrhea is due to excessive weight loss or low body weight, the treatment involves restoring a healthy weight through nutritional counseling, dietary changes, and psychological support.
3. **Structural Abnormalities**: Surgical interventions may be necessary for structural abnormalities that obstruct or affect the reproductive organs. For example, surgery may be performed to remove uterine fibroids or correct abnormalities like an imperforate hymen.
4. **Medications and Treatments**: If amenorrhea is a side effect of certain medications, the healthcare provider may consider adjusting the medication or prescribing alternative options.
5. **Underlying Medical Conditions**: Treatment of chronic medical conditions, such as kidney disease, liver disease, or autoimmune disorders is part of the management.

Chapter 8 **Testes**

The testes have two main functions:

- **Production of sperm** in the seminiferous tubules, with nourishment by *Sertoli cells*, stimulated by pituitary follicle-stimulating hormone (FSH).
- **Production of testosterone** by *Leydig cells* between the seminiferous tubules, stimulated by pituitary luteinizing hormone (LH).

Testosterone

Testosterone is responsible for the development of secondary sexual characteristics (facial hair, deepened voice, increased muscle mass, development of the Adam's apple, male sexual drive [libido], and the growth and development of the male reproduction organs). In women, small amounts of testosterone are produced in the ovaries, adrenal glands, and in peripheral tissues, such as fat and skin. In both men and women, testosterone contributes to bone and muscle strength, brain function, and libido.

Hyperandrogenism

Testosterone excess (*hyperandrogenism*) can occur in either men or women. In women, it may be marked by hirsutism, acne, oily skin, alopecia, and virilization in the form of a deepened voice, increased muscle mass, enlarged clitoris, irregular or absent menstruation, breast atrophy, mood changes, aggressive behavior, hypertension, and decreased fertility. When the source of the excess androgen is polycystic ovary syndrome, there may be ovarian cysts, insulin resistance with a risk for type 2 diabetes, weight gain particularly in the abdominal area, and darkening of the skin folds (*acanthosis nigricans*, which may be due to elevated insulin).

In men, hyperandrogenism similarly may result in acne, alopecia, increased muscle mass, aggressive behavior, and deepened voice. It can also lead to testicular atrophy (decreased LH and FSH secretion from negative feedback to the hypothalamus and pituitary) and reduced fertility.

Hyperandrogenism may arise in:

- Polycystic ovary syndrome
- Congenital adrenal hyperplasia. Commonly, a deficiency in 21-hydroxylase (**Fig. 5-9**) leads to impaired cortisol and aldosterone synthesis and an overproduction of ACTH, which stimulates an excessive production of adrenal androgens.
- Androgen-secreting tumors
- Cushing's syndrome. ACTH stimulation of the adrenal glands can stimulate the production of androgens, such as DHEA and androstenedione, in addition to cortisol. These androgens can be converted to testosterone in the periphery.
- Ovarian hyperthecosis. The theca cells of ovarian follicles normally produce androgens needed for estrogen synthesis, but they produce the androgens excessively in hyperthecosis.

Diagnosis of Hyperandrogenism

The diagnosis of hyperandrogenism may be made through:

- Medical history and exam
- Blood tests:
  - Testosterone level
  - Other hormones for further information as to cause, such as LH, FSH, dehydroepiandrosterone sulfate, 17-hydroxy progesterone, DHEA-S, androstenedione, and sex hormone-binding globulin. (With low levels of the globulin, more free testosterone is available in the bloodstream.)
- Imaging studies (e.g., ultrasound, MRI) to assess ovaries, testes, or adrenal glands for structural abnormalities or tumors that might cause excess testosterone production.

Treatment of Hyperandrogenism

The treatment of hyperandrogenism may include:

- Lifestyle modification (balanced diet, exercise, stress management, adequate sleep)
- Medication:
  - Oral contraceptives. Estrogen and progestin can help regulate hormone levels. They can reduce androgen production by negative feedback that decreases LH and FSH production in the pituitary gland. Decreased LH and FSH results in less testosterone production in the testes and less androgen production in the theca cells of the ovary. Oral contraceptives can improve symptoms like acne and excess hair growth.
  - Anti-androgens. (E.g., *spironolactone* or *cyproterone acetate* can block the effects of androgens.)
  - Insulin-sensitizing agents. *Metformin* for patients with insulin resistance or polycystic ovary syndrome may reduce androgen levels by reducing insulin levels, as insulin can stimulate ovarian androgen synthesis.
- Topical treatment for hirsutism or acne (creams, lotions, or gels containing anti-androgen medications or other agents)
- Laser hair removal or electrolysis
- Ovarian drilling (a laparoscopic procedure in polycystic ovarian syndrome to reduce androgen production and restore ovulation by creating multiple small holes on the ovarian surface)

Hypoandrogenism

Hypoandrogenism may result in:

- Decreased libido
- Erectile dysfunction
- Decreased intensity of orgasm
- Fatigue
- Loss of muscle mass
- Increased body fat. (Loss of muscle mass can lower metabolic rate and increase fat retention.)
- Mood changes and irritability
- Decreased bone density, osteoporosis
- Cognitive changes
- Decreased facial and body hair
- Gynecomastia. (The relative proportion of estrogen in comparison to testosterone increases.)
- Hot flashes in men (may relate to changes in the hypothalamus, which regulates body temperature)

Testosterone deficiency may result from:

- *Primary hypogonadism* (failure of the gonads to produce enough testosterone):
  - Genetic: Klinefelter or Turner syndrome
  - Certain autoimmune diseases, viral infections (mumps), chemotherapy, radiation therapy, or trauma that causes testicular or ovarian damage
- *Secondary hypogonadism*:
  - Hypothalamic or pituitary dysfunction (tumors, pituitary gland disorders, head trauma, with hormonal imbalances)
  - Aging
  - Chronic illnesses (chronic kidney disease, liver disease, HIV/AIDS) may affect the hypothalamic-pituitary-testicular axis.
  - Medications (corticosteroids, opioids, some cancer treatments. Excess corticosteroids can suppress LH secretion, thereby lowering testosterone production. Excess ACTH, though, from a primary pituitary cause, such as an ACTH-secreting tumor, can cause increased androgen production in the adrenals in addition to elevated cortisol.)

Diagnosis of Testosterone Deficiency

The diagnosis of testosterone deficiency may be based on:

- Medical history (decreased libido, erectile dysfunction, fatigue, decreased muscle mass or strength, mood changes, decreased cognitive function)
- Physical exam (decreased body hair, reduced testicular size, gynecomastia)
- Testosterone blood level (usually higher in the morning)
- Other hormone tests. E.g., LH, FSH, estradiol, prolactin (prolactin interferes with hypothalamic GnRH synthesis), and/or sex-hormone-binding globulin levels may provide further insight into potential underlying causes.

- Imaging studies. Ultrasound or MRI of the testes or other structures may reveal tumors or structural abnormalities that could cause testosterone deficiency.

Treatment of Testosterone Deficiency

Treatment of testosterone deficiency includes:

- Testosterone replacement therapy
- Clomiphene (stimulates secretion of GnRH, which leads to elevated LH levels, which stimulates the Leydig cells in the testes to produce more testosterone)
- Lifestyle modifications (adequate diet, exercise, sleep, and stress management)

Chapter 9 **Pituitary Gland and Hypothalamus**

Abnormalities in pituitary gland hormone secretion can occur for different reasons: pituitary tumors, pituitary surgery or radiation, traumatic brain injury, infections/inflammatory conditions (e.g., meningitis, autoimmune diseases), and genetic disorders. One or more hormones can be affected, with symptoms and signs reflective of the particular hormones that are deficient. If a pituitary tumor is large enough, it may compress nearby structures, such as the optic chiasm, where it can cause a bitemporal hemianopia (a lateral field visual loss in each eye) (**Fig. 9-1**).

A pituitary tumor can be actively-secreting, e.g., prolactinomas, growth hormone-secreting tumors, ACTH-secreting tumors, TSH-secreting tumors, gonadotropin-secreting tumors. Or a pituitary tumor may be non-secreting (e.g., chromophobe adenoma). It may be benign (an adenoma – the most common pituitary tumor) or malignant. While a tumor may be benign in the sense of not metastasizing, it can still be highly destructive in damaging the rest of the pituitary gland, particularly if the tumor is large. ACTH or TSH deficiency commonly coincides with a panpituitary defect, where other pituitary hormones are also deficient. Pituitary carcinomas are rare; they can be non-secreting or produce excess hormone. They are treated with surgery, radiation therapy, and chemotherapy.

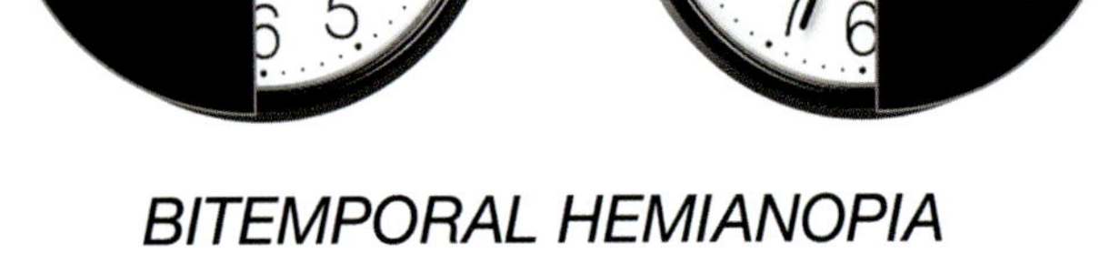

Fig. 9-1. Bitemporal hemianopia (loss of lateral field vision in each eye), characteristic of a lesion to the optic chiasm, as with a large pituitary tumor.

Thyroid-Stimulating Hormone

Thyroid-stimulating hormone (TSH) is secreted by the anterior pituitary gland. It stimulates the thyroid gland to synthesize and release thyroid hormones T3 and T4. Abnormalities in TSH secretion are reflected in abnormalities in thyroid hormone secretion (**Fig. 9-2**). If it is the pituitary tumor which is at fault for the abnormal thyroid hormone secretion, one must consider that there may be additional problems with the secretion of other pituitary hormones that are compromised by the mass effect of the tumor.

The negative feedback of thyroid hormone on the hypothalamus and pituitary gland provides an important way of distinguishing primary from secondary hypothyroidism and hyperthyroidism. For instance, TSH is *increased* in *primary hypothyroidism*, where an underfunctioning thyroid is the main reason for low thyroid hormone and is not suppressing TSH secretion; TSH is decreased, though, in *secondary hypothyroidism* where the pituitary gland is at fault by not secreting TSH to stimulate the thyroid gland (**Fig. 9-2**). Similar reasoning applies for hyperthyroidism (**Fig. 9-2**).

In *tertiary hyperthyroidism/hypothyroidism*, the problem lies with the hypothalamus, which secretes too much or too little thyroid-releasing hormone (TRH), causing the pituitary gland to secrete too much or too little TSH (**Fig. 9-3**). The levels of TSH and thyroid hormone resemble those in secondary hyperthyroidism. Imaging studies (e.g., MRI or CT scan) or an analysis of other hormones that may be deficient can help determine the source of the problem.

Growth Hormone (GH; Somatotropin)

Growth hormone:

- Promotes growth in children and adolescents
- Stimulates cell regeneration
- Stimulates osteoblasts to make bone and increase bone density
- Is important in the metabolism of fats, proteins, and carbohydrates. It breaks down lipids and triglycerides to glycerol and free fatty acids, leading to decreased fat storage.
- Has anti-insulin effects and raises blood glucose levels
- Can stimulate the production and differentiation of immune cells
- Stimulates the production of Insulin-like Growth Factor (IGF-1) in the liver, which has growth-

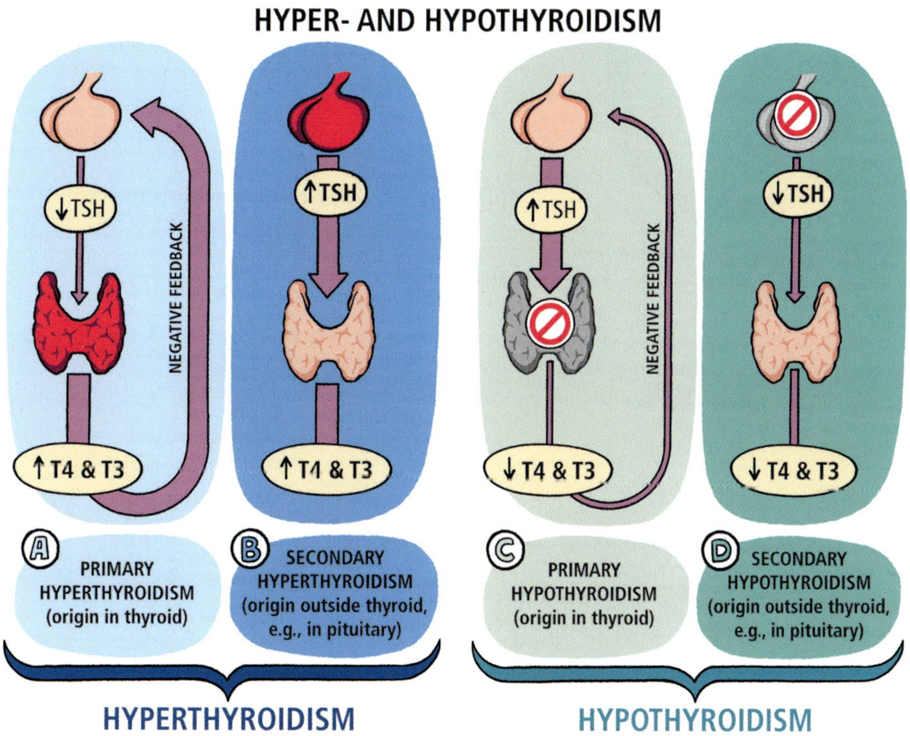

	T4 & T3	TSH
Primary Hyperthyroidism	↑	↓
Secondary Hyperthyroidism	↑	↑
Primary Hypothyroidism	↓	↑
Secondary Hypothyroidism	↓	↓

Fig. 9-2. The combination of thyroid hormone and TSH levels provide a diagnostic clue as to whether a problem with hyperthyroidism or hypothyroidism lies in the thyroid gland or in the brain. (Modified from Berkowitz, A. Clinical Pathophysiology Made Ridiculously Simple. Medmaster.)

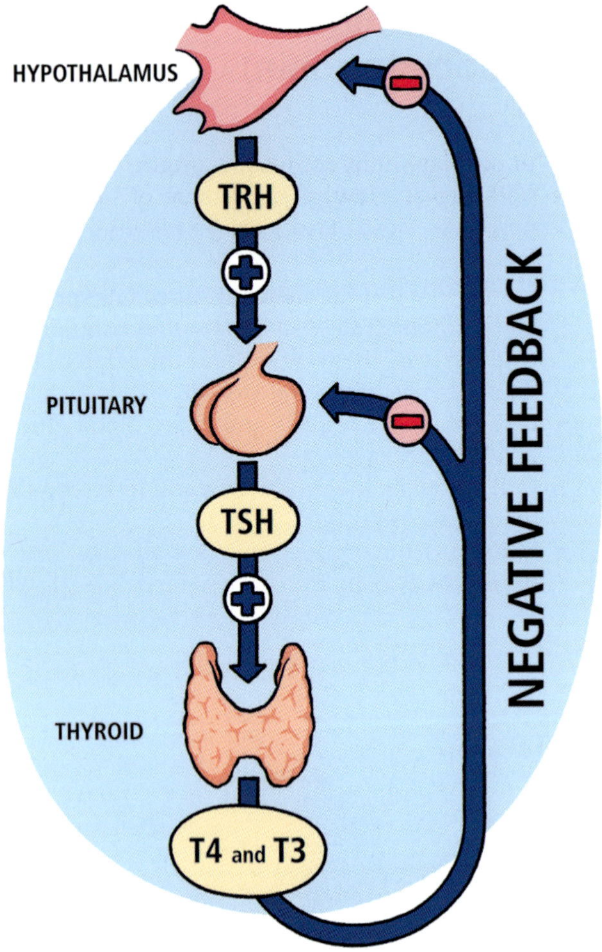

Fig. 9-3. Tertiary hyperthyroidism. The hypothalamus releases excess thyroid-releasing hormone (TRH), which stimulates excess secretion of pituitary secretion of TSH. Feedback of excess T4 and T3 inhibits both TRH and TSH secretion, but not enough to prevent hyperthyroidism. (Modified from Berkowitz, A. Clinical Pathophysiology Made Ridiculously Simple. Medmaster.)

stimulating effects like GH but, unlike GH, has insulin-like effects, promoting glucose uptake in muscle and fat tissue and lowering blood glucose

- Augments the effects of LH and FSH on the gonads, aiding in ovulation and spermatogenesis
- Helps maintain a healthy balance between muscle and fat tissues

Excess Growth Hormone

Signs of Growth Hormone Excess

The effects of excess growth hormone include:

- *Acromegaly* in adults (enlarged nose, protruding jaw, thickened lips, widely spaced teeth, enlarged hands and feet [**Fig. 9-4**], increased shoe and ring size, enlarged hands and fingers, enlarged bones and joints, arthritis-like symptoms, enlarged heart, liver and spleen, menstrual irregularities, erectile dysfunction, headaches, vision problems, and other hormonal imbalances). Acromegaly may produce hypogonadism through compression of a pituitary tumor mass on pituitary gonadotropic cells.
- *Gigantism* in children. This may be marked by excessive height, rapid growth, cardiomegaly, hepatomegaly, renomegaly, joint pain and limited mobility, scoliosis or kyphosis, headaches, and vision problems. It may cause delayed sexual development, due in part to feedback by GH to the pituitary, which can suppress the release of GnRH and gonadotropins such as LH and FSH. Gigantism transitions into acromegaly at the end of puberty when the growth plates close.

Causes of Growth Hormone Excess

- Pituitary adenomas or hyperplasia. Multiple Endocrine Neoplasia type 1, McCune-Albright syndrome and Carney complex arise from genetic mutations that may include growth hormone-secreting pituitary tumors.
- Ectopic GH-secreting tumors (e.g., in lung, pancreas)
- Neuroendocrine tumors that secrete GH
- Exogenous use of GH by body builders

Diagnosis of Growth Hormone Excess

- History and physical suggestive of acromegaly or gigantism.
- GH and IGF-1 levels elevated. (Excess GH stimulates hepatic secretion of insulin-like growth factor, which causes most of the clinical manifestations of acromegaly.)
- Oral glucose tolerance test (normally suppresses GH release, but GH may remain elevated in

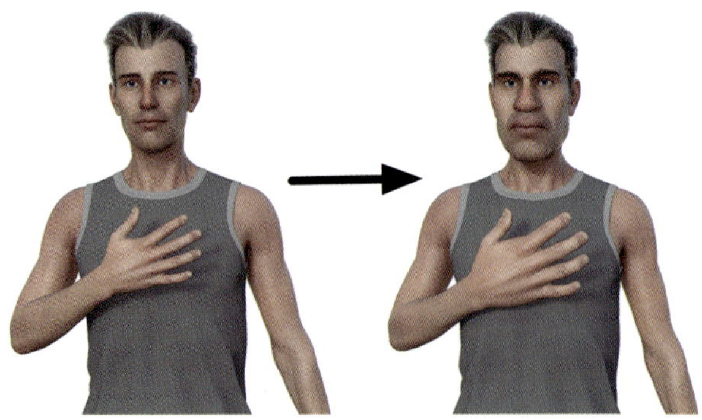

Fig. 9-4. Acromegaly

acromegaly and gigantism, usually due to a non-suppressing pituitary adenoma)

- Imaging studies (MRI, CT of pituitary) to detect a pituitary adenoma
- Visual field testing. (The pituitary gland lies near the optic chiasm and optic nerves, which may be compromised. Bitemporal hemianopia **[Fig. 9-1]** is characteristic of an optic chiasm lesion.)
- Evaluate other hormones that might be involved, e.g., prolactin, thyroid hormones, and adrenal hormones. Prolactin may be elevated in addition to GH when a pituitary tumor damages the pituitary stalk. This interrupts the delivery of dopamine (which inhibits prolactin secretion) from the hypothalamus, leading to increased prolactin together with the increased GH levels.

Treatment of Growth Hormone Excess

- Surgery (removal of the GH-secreting pituitary adenoma, generally by a transsphenoidal approach through the nasal cavity)
- Medication:
  - Somatostatin analogs. *Octreotide* and *lanreotide* suppress GH secretion.
  - Dopamine agonists (e.g., *cabergoline, bromocriptine*). Dopamine normally inhibits GH secretion, as does somatostatin.
  - Growth hormone receptor antagonists, e.g., *pegvisomant* (blocks the action of GH on target tissues, including the liver's production of IGF-1)
- Radiation therapy if surgery and medications are not effective or feasible

Growth Hormone Deficiency

Signs of Growth Hormone Deficiency

- Children: Short stature, slow growth rate, delayed puberty, increased body fat (GH normally breaks down fat for energy), immature appearance
- Adults: Fatigue, decreased muscle mass, increased body fat, reduced bone density (osteoporosis), increased LDL cholesterol, decreased HDL cholesterol

Causes of Growth Hormone Deficiency

- Damage to the pituitary gland or hypothalamus (craniopharyngioma, pituitary adenoma, pituitary surgery, radiation, trauma, genetic disorders, e.g., Turner syndrome, Prader-Willi syndrome). Craniopharyngioma is the most common tumor in children that affects the pituitary gland.
- Idiopathic

Diagnosis of Growth Hormone Deficiency

- GH stimulation tests: Arginine, clonidine, glucagon, and insulin normally stimulate release of GH. If they don't, this suggests GH deficiency of pituitary or hypothalamic origin.
- IGF-1 levels (low) is a measure of GH activity. IGF-1 measurement is more reliable than GH measurement since GH is secreted in pulses and levels can vary greatly throughout the day.
- Assess other pituitary hormones that may be affected.

Treatment of Growth Hormone Deficiency

The treatment of growth hormone deficiency is mainly by growth hormone replacement. Treatment with GH is contraindicated in patients with active malignancy due to concern that it might stimulate the growth and spread of cancer cells.

FSH and LH

Follicle-stimulating hormone (FSH) and **luteinizing hormone (LH)** are important in both males and females. Both hormones are produced in the anterior pituitary gland, and the release of both is stimulated by gonadotropin-releasing hormone (GnRH) from the hypothalamus. FSH and LH are commonly measured together when evaluating reproductive health.

In *females*, pituitary **FSH** stimulates the growth of ovarian follicles and their secretion of estradiol, which supports the development of the uterine endometrium in preparation for pregnancy. **LH** triggers the release of the mature egg from the ovarian follicle during ovulation and the formation of the **corpus luteum** from the follicle. The corpus luteum secretes **progesterone** to maintain the uterine lining for potential implantation of a fertilized egg and helps maintain pregnancy if fertilization occurs.

In *males*, **FSH** stimulates spermatogenesis while **LH** stimulates testosterone production.

FSH and LH Deficiency

In females, FSH and LH deficiency can lead to anovulation, disrupted menstrual cycles, infertility and hypoestrogenism.

In males, FSH and LH deficiency may result in delayed or absent puberty, testicular atrophy, decreased sperm, and infertility.

Causes of FSH and LH deficiency include:

- Pituitary or hypothalamic dysfunction
  - Destructive pituitary tumors
  - *Kallman syndrome* (anosmia and impaired GnRH-producing neurons)

- *Sheehan syndrome* (postpartum pituitary necrosis)
- Autoimmune disorders of the hypothalamus or pituitary gland

- Secreting ovarian or testicular tumors can, by negative feedback to the pituitary, decrease FSH and LH levels.
- Chronic stress

Diagnosis of FSH and LH Deficiency

- History and physical (menstrual irregularities, fertility issues, decreased libido)
- Blood tests:
  - LH, FSH, estradiol (females) and testosterone (males). Low LH/FSH levels may indicate primary LH/FSH deficiency. High levels in the presence of gonadal insufficiency suggest primary gonadal failure with feedback to the pituitary to increase LH/FSH secretion.
- Measurement of other pituitary hormones may help determine whether the problem lies in hypothalamic or pituitary dysfunction.
- Imaging studies (MRI or CT of the hypothalamus or pituitary gland)
- *GnRH (gonadotropin-releasing hormone) stimulation test.* (Low FSH and LH levels after GnRH administration may suggest a primary pituitary deficiency in FSH and LH secretion. An increased response suggests that the problem may lie in the hypothalamus' inability to secrete GnRH.)
- Genetic testing

Treatment of FSH and LH Deficiency

- Sex hormone replacement (estrogen or testosterone)
- GnRH therapy to stimulate the pituitary gland to produce LH and FSH, especially when fertility is the issue.
- Hormone replacement (with FSH and LH)
- *Clomiphene* stimulates the hypothalamus to secrete GnRH, which stimulates LH and FSH secretion. GnRh agonists like *leuprolide* can stimulate the pituitary gland to release LH and FSH; dopamine agonists like *bromocriptine* or *cabergoline* reduce prolactin (which normally inhibits the release of GnRH) and may increase and normalize LH and FSH levels.
- Human chorionic gonadotropin (hCG) can mimic the action of LH and is a treatment used for infertility in women to stimulate ovulation. In men, it can be used to stimulate the Leydig cells of the testes to produce testosterone.
- Surgery, radiation, or medication to manage a pituitary or hypothalamic tumor
- Assisted reproductive techniques (in vitro fertilization; intrauterine insemination)

Prolactin

Prolactin has numerous functions throughout the body, but it is usually thought of in reference to lactation. It stimulates growth of the breast ductal system in pregnancy and stimulates the mammary glands to produce milk during breastfeeding. Prolactin also interacts with other hormones (it inhibits the secretion of GnRH), contributes to the regulation of the menstrual cycle, and has effects on insulin sensitivity and fat metabolism, bone health, fluid and electrolyte balance, and the immune system.

Prolactin Excess (Hyperprolactinemia)

Symptoms and Signs of Prolactin Excess

- Women: Irregular menstrual periods or amenorrhea from inhibition of GnRH secretion by the hypothalamus; galactorrhea in non-pregnant women, infertility
- Men: Erectile dysfunction; decreased testosterone levels by inhibiting GnRH secretion; decreased libido, and sometimes gynecomastia (from decreased testosterone/estrogen ratio)
- In both: Headaches, vision changes (with pituitary prolactinoma)
- Decreased bone density through decreased secretion of GnRH; decreased GnRH leads to decreased production of estrogen in women and testosterone in men, which are important in maintaining bone density.

Causes of Prolactin Excess

- Prolactinoma of the pituitary gland (the most common cause; prolactinomas are the most common pituitary tumors in adults and are more common in women.)
- Pregnancy
- Pituitary damage that interrupts the dopamine pathways, which normally inhibit prolactin secretion.
- Medications that directly or indirectly block dopamine pathways or receptors: some anti-psychoticdrugs(e.g.,*risperidone,haloperidol,SSRIs*), antidepressants (e.g., *tricyclic antidepressants*), blood pressure medications (*verapamil*), cocaine, heroin, and alcohol
- Estrogen therapy can cause hyperprolactinemia because estrogen stimulates the pituitary gland to produce prolactin, as seen in pregnancy, where estrogen levels are high.
- Hypothyroidism. (Thyroid-releasing hormone elevation, from feeback by reduced thyroid hormone, stimulates both TSH and prolactin secretion.)

- Chronic kidney disease (impaired prolactin clearance)
- Idiopathic

Diagnosis of Prolactin Excess

- Blood tests:
  - Serum prolactin levels
  - Urine or serum hCG test for pregnancy
  - Other hormones - TSH, estradiol (in females), testosterone (males) for associated deficits
- Imaging studies (MRI of the pituitary gland to determine if there is a prolactinoma)
- Thyroid function tests (TSH, thyroid hormones). There is an association between hyper-prolactinemia and thyroid dysfunction, particularly hypothyroidism, since decreased thyroid hormone, apart from stimulating TSH secretion can also stimulate prolactin secretion.
- Other hormonal tests may also provide helpful information (e.g., pituitary hormone levels, assessment of gonadal function).

Treatment of Prolactin Excess

- Medication: Dopamine agonists, e.g., *bromocriptine* or *cabergoline* reduce prolactin secretion and can shrink a prolactin-secreting tumor. *Dopamine agonists are the first-line treatment for prolactinoma.*
- Surgery if needed for a pituitary tumor
- Radiation
- Management of associated conditions: Hormone replacement for hypothyroidism or specific treatment for polycystic ovary syndrome. (Some women with PCOS may have elevated prolactin levels).

Prolactin Deficiency

Symptoms and Signs of Prolactin Deficiency

- Inability to produce breast milk
- Irregular periods
- Decreased libido
- Infertility

Causes of Prolactin Deficiency

- Sheehan's postpartum pituitary necrosis
- Pituitary tumors (nonfunctioning)
- Pituitary surgery, radiation
- Medications - dopamine agonists, e.g., *bromocriptine, cabergoline, pergolide*. Dopamine normally inhibits prolactin secretion.

Diagnosis of Prolactin Deficiency

- Blood tests (prolactin level, TSH, FSH, GH, estradiol, testosterone)
- *Thyrotropin-releasing hormone (TRH) stimulation test*. Normally, TRH simulates an increase in the levels of both TSH and prolactin. If it doesn't, this implies a dysfunction of the pituitary gland.
- *Metoclopramide stimulation test.* Metoclopramide is a dopamine receptor antagonist that stimulates the release of prolactin from the pituitary. If it doesn't, this suggests a pituitary gland problem.
- Imaging studies (CT or MRI of the hypothalamus and pituitary gland)
- Genetic testing (mutations that relate to prolactin production)

Treatment of Prolactin Deficiency

Prolactin deficiency can be treated with prolactin hormone replacement, as well as by symptomatic management and treating the underlying condition. E.g., hypothalamic/pituitary dysfunction may be approached with surgery, radiation, or medication.

Antidiuretic Hormone

Antidiuretic hormone (ADH; vasopressin) and oxytocin are produced in the hypothalamus but are stored in and released from hypothalamic nerve fibers that end in the posterior pituitary gland (**Fig. 1-3**). ADH increases water reabsorption in the medullary collecting duct of the kidney, which can increase blood volume and blood pressure. ADH also can raise blood pressure by vasoconstriction. The "antidiuretic" name ADH refers to the ability of ADH to reabsorb water. The alternate name "vasopressin" refers to the ability of ADH to vasoconstrict.

The main stimulus to ADH secretion by the hypothalamus is an increase in concentration of sodium (the main extracellular ion) and serum osmolality. The hypothalamus responds by releasing ADH to increase renal water reabsorption. ADH secretion is also stimulated by low blood pressure, detected by baroreceptors in the carotid and aortic sinuses, which signal the hypothalamus to secrete ADH and also stimulate the sympathetic nervous system to increase blood pressure (**Figs. 6-1** and **6-2**).

The interaction of ADH with other body parameters that control blood pressure is discussed in **Chapter 6** (*Hypertension*).

Syndrome of Inappropriate Antidiuretic Hormone Secretion (SIADH)

SIADH results in the excess renal reabsorption of water, causing not only water retention and decreased urine output, but hyponatremia from blood dilution, an osmotic imbalance. Water then moves intracellularly, leading to cellular swelling, which may cause cerebral edema, with symptoms ranging from mild headache and nausea to confusion, seizures, stupor and coma when severe. *Too rapid* correction of a severe hyponatremia can lead to another severe condition, *osmotic demyelination syndrome* (*ODS; central pontine myelinosis*) from the rapid osmotic change. ODS can present with confusion, coma, quadriparesis, difficulty swallowing or speaking, cranial nerve defects, and, in severe cases, the "locked-in" syndrome, where the patient is conscious but cannot move.

The causes of SIADH include:

- Ectopic ADH production (from a small cell lung cancer or other lung tumors, head and neck tumors, thymoma, pancreatic tumors, certain brain tumors, GI or prostate cancer, or lymphoma)
- Medications: Some antidepressants, antiepileptic, antipsychotic, narcotic, and chemotherapeutic drugs can enhance the release or effect of ADH.
- Inflammatory lung diseases, e.g., pneumonia and COPD, may result in excess ADH production by the hypothalamic / pituitary axis.
- Trauma to the brain; diseases affecting the pituitary gland or hypothalamus
- Volume depletion stimulating ADH secretion
- Potentiation of the renal tubular effect of ADH
- Rare hereditary conditions
- Idiopathic

Diagnosis of SIADH

- Patients with SIADH generally do not have peripheral edema. The excess water retention tends to remain in the circulatory system rather than escaping into the peripheral tissues.
- Is the patient taking any medications that may cause SIADH?
- Blood tests: serum sodium concentration (low), serum osmolality (typically low).
- Urine sodium concentration (typically elevated), and urine osmolality (typically elevated)
- Rule out other causes of hyponatremia; e.g., excess water intake, congestive heart failure, liver or kidney disease, adrenal insufficiency, excessive sweating, or drugs that can cause hyponatremia).
- MRI or CT scan of the brain may detect abnormalities associated with SIADH.
- Correction of hyponatremia by fluid restriction helps confirm the diagnosis of SIADH since the primary issue is water retention and fluid overload rather than a lack of sodium.

Treatment of SIADH

- Fluid and water restriction
- Hypertonic sodium chloride for severe symptoms (e.g., seizures, altered mental status)
- Loop diuretics, e.g., furosemide, inhibit water reabsorption.
- Vasopressin receptor antagonists (**vaptans**, e.g., *conivaptan* or *tolvaptan*) antagonize the action of ADH.
- *Demeclocycline* acts on the renal collecting ducts to decrease their receptiveness to ADH, by a different mechanism than the vaptans.
- Monitor and correct sodium imbalances.
- Treat the underlying cause and symptoms.

Diabetes Insipidus

Diabetes insipidus is a disorder caused by insufficient secretion of ADH by the posterior pituitary gland. It is characterized by the excretion of large volumes of very dilute urine (polyuria), and consequent excessive thirst (polydipsia), frequently along with hypernatremia from the water loss, which could be as much as 20 liters / day in severe cases. Symptoms of hypernatremia from rapid dehydration may range from weakness to coma and seizures.

Diabetes insipidus (DI) can be caused by either decreased ADH or a failure of the kidney to respond to it:

- *Central diabetes insipidus* (from head trauma, tumor, infection, brain surgery, granulomatous disease, or cerebrovascular disease that damages the hypothalamus or pituitary gland) can result in decreased ADH secretion.
- *Nephrogenic diabetes insipidus* occurs when the kidney doesn't respond to ADH because of a genetic mutation or an acquired condition such as chronic kidney disease, certain medications (e.g., lithium, loop diuretics, some antibiotics), or high levels of calcium in the blood (high calcium can inhibit the channels in the kidney that reabsorb water) (**Fig. 9-5**)
- Gestational diabetes insipidus can occur from breakdown of ADH by the placenta in pregnancy.
- Primary polydipsia (**Fig. 9-6**) can mimic diabetes insipidus. It causes polyuria and a dilute urine and suppresses ADH secretion. However, it tends toward hyponatremia, rather than the hypernatremia often found in diabetes insipidus.
- Genetic conditions can be responsible for either central diabetes insipidus (*Familial Neurohypophyseal Diabetes Insipidus; Wolfram Syndrome*) or nephrogenic diabetes insipidus (*X-linked Nephrogenic Diabetes Insipidus; Autosomal Recessive and Dominant Nephrogenic Diabetes Insipidus*).

Diagnosis of Diabetes Insipidus

- High plasma hyperosmolality, including hypernatremia, if thirst does not replenish sufficient water.
- Dilute urine

- Polyuria (can also occur in diabetes mellitus, intrinsic renal disease, or excess fluid intake, certain medications (e.g., diuretics), urinary tract inflammation, pregnancy, and high calcium levels)
- Blood test, where available, for ADH levels in blood (decreased)
- **Water deprivation test**. After water deprivation for about 4-5 hours (not done when the patient is already hypernatremic), the patient continues to produce large amounts of dilute urine with diabetes insipidus, as opposed to primary polydipsia.
- **ADH stimulation test**. After water deprivation, the patient is given synthetic ADH (*desmopressin*). If the kidneys respond by concentrating the urine, it suggests that the kidneys are functioning properly and the problem lies with ADH secretion (central diabetes insipidus). If the kidneys do not respond, it suggests a problem with the kidney response to ADH rather than the amount of ADH (nephrogenic diabetes insipidus) (**Fig. 9-5**).
- Large amounts of sugar in the urine in a patient with excess thirst and polyuria may be a sign of type 1 or type 2 diabetes mellitus rather than diabetes insipidus.
- An MRI scan can check for abnormality in the hypothalamus or pituitary gland.
- Genetic testing

Treatment of Diabetes Insipidus

- Drink water to prevent dehydration.
- *Desmopressin*, a synthetic form of ADH, can be given for central diabetes insipidus.
- In nephrogenic diabetes insipidus, where desmopressin does not help, NSAIDs plus thiazide diuretics can be helpful. Thiazides increase sodium excretion and paradoxically reduce urine volume in nephrogenic diabetes insipidus. NSAIDs can enhance the action of thiazides.
- Correct the underlying cause.

Hypothalamic Releasing Hormones

The hypothalamus produces ADH and oxytocin, which reach the posterior pituitary by nerve axon extensions (**Fig. 1-3**). It also produces **releasing hormones**, which are secreted in variably-timed pulses, in some cases in a circadian rhythm, that reach the anterior pituitary gland by the pituitary venous portal circulation. Releasing hormones affect the synthesis and release of the anterior pituitary gland hormones. The releasing hormones include:

- **Gonadotropin-releasing hormone (GnRH)** stimulates the release of pituitary FSH and LH. Low frequency pulses stimulate mainly FSH release, while high frequency pulses stimulate LH release.
- **Corticotropin-releasing hormone (CRH)** stimulates the release of pituitary ACTH.
- **Growth hormone-releasing hormone (GHRH; somatotropin)** stimulates the release of pituitary growth hormone.
- **Prolactin-inhibiting hormone (PIH; dopamine)** – *inhibits* the release of pituitary prolactin.

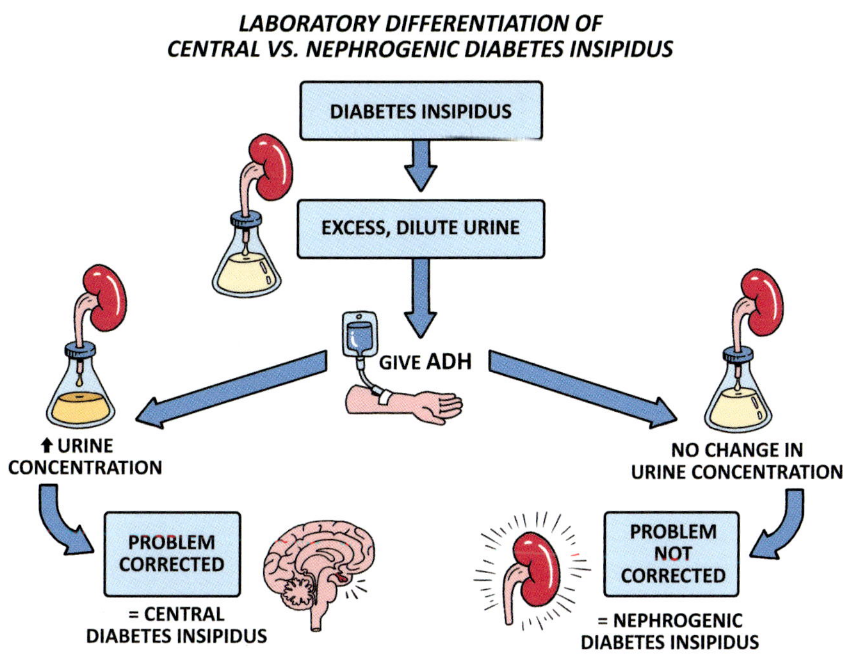

Fig. 9-5.

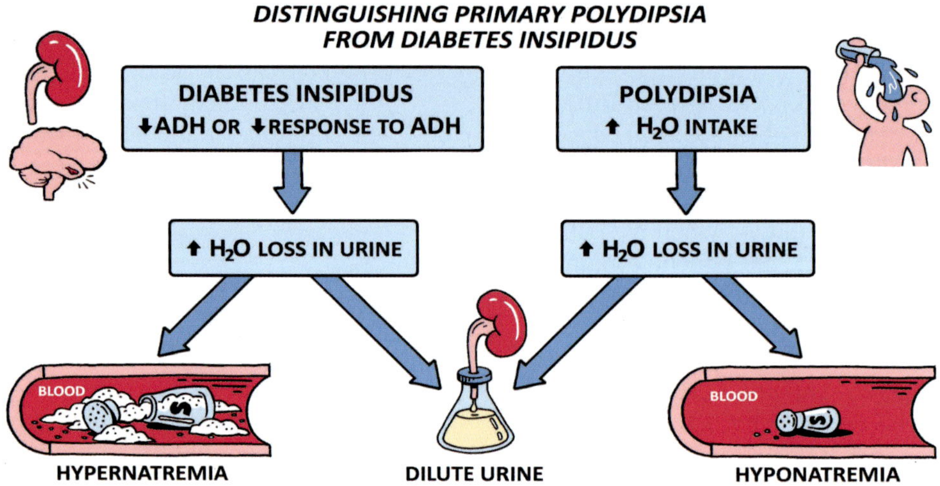

Fig. 9-6.

- **Thyroid-releasing hormone (TRH)** stimulates the release of pituitary thyroid-stimulating hormone (TSH).
- **Somatostatin-inhibiting hormone** is in a sense an "anti-releasing" hormone. In the pituitary, it mainly inhibits the release of growth hormone (GH) and thyroid-stimulating hormone (TSH).

The same feedback mechanisms from the periphery that directly affect the secretion of pituitary hormones also affect the secretion of the corresponding hypothalamic releasing factors (**Fig. 1-3**). Over- or under-secretion of releasing factors is reflected in corresponding deficits in their pituitary hormone counterparts.

Determining whether a hormonal problem originates in the pituitary gland or the hypothalamus can be approached in several ways:

- MRI imaging can visualize the pituitary gland and hypothalamus to help determine where the problem lies.
- Sometimes the response to specific treatments can point to the source of the problem. For instance, treating with a releasing hormone could bypass a hypothalamic issue, while it wouldn't resolve a pituitary defect.
- Some hypothalamic disorders can affect functions like body temperature regulation, appetite, thirst, and sleep patterns due to the hypothalamus' control over these functions. These symptoms might not be prominent in isolated pituitary disorders.
- Hypothalamic defects are more likely to affect multiple hormones than do pituitary defects.
- Hormone level comparisons may provide a clue. For instance, a high TSH / high TRH would suggest a hypothalamic cause of hyperthyroidism, while a high TSH, low TRH would suggest a pituitary cause, since the resulting high thyroid hormone levels feed back to inhibit the hypothalamus.
- Sometimes genetic testing may provide information about inherited disorders affecting the hypothalamus or pituitary.

Pineal Gland

The pineal gland is an unpaired structure near the center of the brain. Contrary to Descartes, the pineal gland is not the center of consciousness, as is clear from the persistence of consciousness in patients who have had a pinealoma removed.

Although the pineal gland is not part of the hypothalamus, it does receive indirect neural connections from the suprachiasmatic nucleus of the hypothalamus as part of the regulation of the circadian rhythm (**Fig. 9-7**). The pineal gland secretes the hormone *melatonin*, which promotes sleep. Its release is stimulated by darkness and suppressed by light. Melatonin is commonly used to treat insomnia, whereas difficulty in awakening on time can be treated by turning on the light.

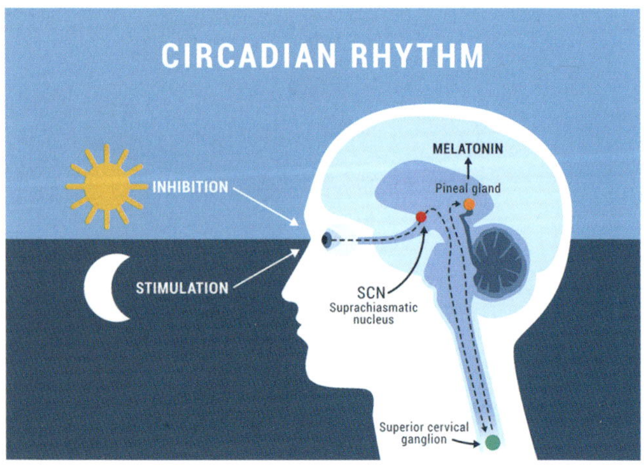

Fig. 9-7. Melatonin secretion by the pineal gland.

Chapter 10 **Heart**

Atrial Natriuretic Peptide (ANP)

Atrial Natriuretic Peptide is a hormone produce by cardiac atrial muscle cells (myocytes) in response to atrial stretch, which usually is caused by increased blood volume or elevated blood pressure. *ANP helps reduce blood volume and blood pressure* by several mechanisms:

- ANP promotes the excretion of sodium in the urine (natriuresis), with water following the sodium, leading to increased urine volume and decreased blood pressure.
- ANP relaxes vascular smooth muscle, causing vasodilation and reduced blood pressure.
- ANP inhibits the secretion of renin from the kidney, thereby reducing the activity of the renin-angiotensin-aldosterone system, causing more natriuresis and vasodilation.
- ANP inhibits aldosterone secretion from the adrenal gland.
- ANP counteracts pathological hypertrophy of the heart in response to high blood pressure.

B-Type Natriuretic Peptide (BNP)

B-type Natriuretic Peptide (BNP) is produced in ventricular muscles cells, where it is released in response to ventricular stretch. It does similar things as ANP, but also, to a greater extent than ANP, inhibits cardiac hypertrophy in response to chronic heart failure. BNP, which is more stable than ANP, is used as a biomarker for assessing the severity of heart failure.

Chapter 11 **Liver**

The liver has numerous metabolic functions, including detoxification and the synthesis of various molecules. While it is not typically recognized as an endocrine gland, the liver does produce and release certain hormones and signaling molecules. These include:

- **Insulin-like Growth Factor 1 (IGF-1)**
- **Thrombopoietin (TPO)**
- **Hepcidin**
- **Angiotensinogen**

Insulin-like Growth Factor 1 (IGF-1)

The liver synthesizes and secretes **IGF-1 (Somatomedin C)** in response to growth hormone (GH) from the pituitary gland.

- IGF-1 plays a vital role in promoting tissue growth and development, especially during childhood and adolescence.
- IGF-1 enhances muscle growth by promoting protein synthesis and the proliferation and differentiation of muscle cells, including muscle repair and regeneration.
- IGF-1 also promotes glucose uptake in tissues and releases fatty acids from adipose tissue for conversion to acetyl-CoA for energy. This can provide an advantage in energy utilization during prolonged physical activity. For these reasons, IGF-1 has been used as a performance-enhancing substance (considered doping, which is banned by professional sports). It also can lead to health problems, including an increased risk of certain cancers, metabolic imbalances, and cardiovascular issues.

While growth hormone (GH) and IGF-1 have synergistic effects in promoting tissue growth and development, they have opposite effects on glucose metabolism. GH tends to increase blood glucose levels, while IGF-1 decreases blood glucose by enhancing glucose uptake into cells. GH (and sometimes IGF-1) can be used to treat specific instances of growth failure in children.

The concentration of IGF-1 is relatively stable throughout the day, unlike GH, which is secreted in pulses. This makes IGF-1 a valuable tool in more accurately detecting deficiency or excess in GH secretion.

Insulin-like Growth Factor-Binding Protein 1 (IGFBP-1) is a protein that binds to IGF-1, modulating its actions and availability in the bloodstream. While it can prolong the half-life of IGF-1 in the circulation it can also inhibit its interaction with IGF receptors.

Thrombopoietin (TPO)

TPO is a hormone produced by the liver and other tissues, such as the kidney. It stimulates the production and maturation of platelets, which are important for blood clotting. Thrombopoietin receptor agonists (e.g., *etrombopag, romiplostim, avatrombopag*) can be used therapeutically to increase platelet production when platelets are abnormally low.

Hepcidin

Hepcidin plays a crucial role in iron metabolism. It reduces iron absorption in the intestines and prevents iron release into the blood from liver hepatocytes, thereby lowering blood iron levels. Excessively high levels of iron in the blood (as well as inflammation) stimulate hepcidin production, while low iron levels suppress it, ensuring that iron levels are kept within a healthy range. Too much hepcidin can lead to iron-deficiency anemia, while too little can lead to iron overload disorders like hemochromatosis, which can damage organs. The iron-deficiency anemia can be treated with iron supplementation. The excess iron in hemochromatosis can be treated by phlebotomy, iron chelation, or a low-iron diet, as the body normally does not have a good way of getting rid of excess iron. Treating the underlying inflammatory or infectious conditions can help normalize hepcidin levels.

Angiotensinogen

Angiotensinogen is a glycoprotein precursor to the hormone angiotensin in the renin-angiotensin-aldosterone system, which helps regulate blood pressure and fluid volume (**Fig. 12-1**).

Chapter 12 **Kidney**

Renin

Renin is an enzyme produced by the juxtaglomerular cells of the kidney (**Fig. 5-8A** and **5-8B**). Some would also call renin a hormone since it circulates in the bloodstream and is important in activating hormone production in the renin-angiotensin-aldosterone system (**Fig. 12-1**):

- When blood pressure drops, the kidneys release *renin*.
- *Renin* cleaves liver *angiotensinogen* to form *angiotensin I*, which is still relatively inactive.
- *Angiotensin I* is converted to *angiotensin II*, an active molecule, by angiotensin-converting enzyme (ACE), found mainly in the lungs. Angiotensin II has important functions in maintaining blood pressure and fluid volume:
    - Angiotensin II is a vasoconstrictor, causing blood pressure to rise.
    - Angiotensin II stimulates sympathetic outflow from the brainstem and hypothalamus.
    - Angiotensin II stimulates antidiuretic hormone (ADH) release by the pituitary gland. ADH acts on the kidneys to retain water and maintain fluid volume and blood pressure.
    - Angiotensin II stimulates the release of adrenal catecholamines with consequent increase in heart rate and contractility.
    - Angiotensin II stimulates the adrenal gland to release aldosterone, which causes the kidneys to retain sodium and water, further increasing blood pressure (**Fig. 12-1**). Angiotensin II itself simulates sodium and water reabsorption in the renal tubules.
    - Angiotensin II stimulates thirst, encouraging fluid intake.

Further details about the interaction of renin with the other mechanisms of blood pressure control may be found in **Chapter 6** (*Hypertension*).

Hyperreninemia

Excess renin (hyperreninemia) can cause hypertension and sodium and water retention.

The potential causes of excess renin include:

- Renal artery stenosis. Decreased blood flow to the kidneys stimulates renin secretion.
- Renin-secreting tumors
- Chronic kidney disease. (Renin release increases when there is reduced renal blood flow and GFR.)
- Heart failure. (Decreased blood flow causes the release of renin to maintain blood pressure and perfusion.)
- Liver cirrhosis with ascites. (The body senses a reduction in effective circulating volume.)
- Nonsteroidal anti-inflammatory drugs (NSAIDs) that block prostaglandin production can indirectly stimulate renin release. (Prostaglandins produced in the kidney normally inhibit the release of renin.)

Renin-angiotensin-aldosterone system

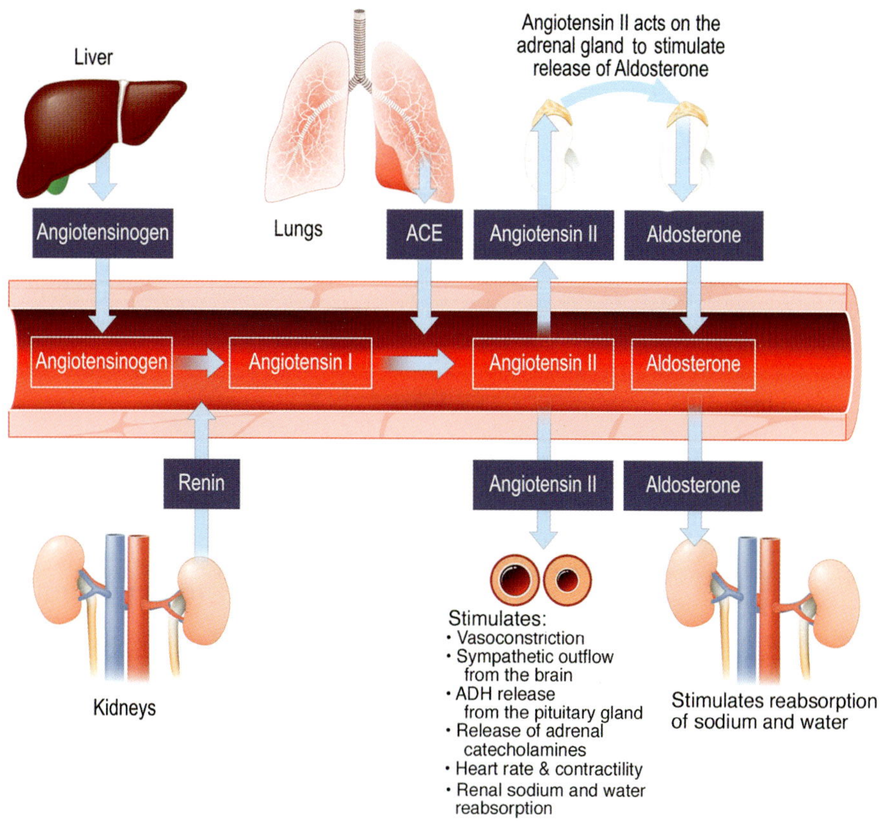

Fig. 12-1. The renin-angiotensin-aldosterone system.

Finding the cause for renin excess may involve measuring renin and aldosterone levels, imaging (e.g., renal ultrasound, CT for renal artery stenosis or renal mass), and liver and renal function tests. In *primary hyperaldosteronism*, where there is an aldosterone-producing adenoma, aldosterone levels will be high, but renin levels will be suppressed due to negative feedback on kidney secretion of renin. The "aldosterone/renin ratio" will be high. In *secondary hyperaldosteronism* due to excess renin secretion, both renin and aldosterone levels will be high, since increased renin stimulates the renin-angiotensin-aldosterone system to produce aldosterone.

Treatment for renin excess includes:

- Addressing the underlying cause (e.g., renal artery stenosis, heart failure, liver disease)
- Antihypertensive medications
- Sodium restriction and fluid management

Hyporeninemia

The signs of primary renin *deficiency* (hyporeninemia) include hypotension, hyponatremia/hyperkalemia (from decreased aldosterone), and polyuria/dehydration (less fluid reabsorption). The cause of the renin deficiency may be chronic kidney disease with impaired renin production, primary aldosteronism (which suppresses renin production, but which will cause hypertension), or genetic. The diagnosis can be confirmed by blood tests for renin and aldosterone, imaging of the kidneys and adrenal glands, and in some cases, genetic testing.

The **treatment** for primary renin deficiency includes:

- Increased salt intake
- Hydration
- Medications, e.g., *fludrocortisone* (for its aldosterone-like effect), *midodrine* (a vasoconstrictor) for hypotension.
- Monitoring of electrolytes

Erythropoietin (EPO)

Erythropoietin (EPO) is a hormone mainly produced by the kidneys; the liver produces a small amount. When oxygen levels drop, the kidney senses this and releases more EPO. EPO stimulates the production of red blood cells in the bone marrow and accelerates their maturation.

Erythropoietin excess results in:

- An abnormal increase in red blood cells (*polycythemia*)
- Splenomegaly from an attempt by the spleen to clear the excess red blood cells (RBCs) or produce new ones
- Hypertension (resistance to blood flow)
- Increased risk of blood clotting

An excess of erythropoietin may arise from:

- Hypoxia
- An erythropoietin-secreting renal cell tumor
- Liver disease (reduced blood oxygenation from a porto-caval shunt; decreased clearance of EPO; an erythropoietin-secreting hepatocellular tumor)
- Genetic conditions that cause excess EPO production or increased sensitivity to low oxygen

Polycythemia

Primary polycythemia (polycythemia vera) is a form of blood cancer in which the bone marrow intrinsically produces too many red blood cells. **Secondary polycythemia** is a response to other factors, such as low oxygen or an erythropoietin-secreting tumor, which cause an increase in EPO.

Diagnosis of Polycythemia

Polycythemia can be confirmed by an increased RBC count and hematocrit. The cause can be clarified by:

- Blood EPO measurement. If high, consider high altitude, smoking, and chronic hypoxia. Low or normal levels are more consistent with a primary polycythemia.
- Oxygen saturation levels in arterial blood or pulse oximetry
- Imaging studies (renal ultrasound, CT, MRI for tumors or other abnormality)
- Bone marrow evaluation, which can differentiate *polycythemia vera* from secondary polycythemia from EPO excess

Treatment of Polycythemia:

- The treatment of polycythemia includes: Addressing the cause (e.g., renal cell carcinoma, liver disease, hypoxia, polycythemia vera)
- Phlebotomy
- Medication to suppress EPO or red cell production:
  - *Hydroxyurea* can decrease RBC production.
  - *JAK 2 inhibitors* inhibit the mutant enzyme responsible for erythrocytosis in certain myeloproliferative neoplasms.
- Fluid management to prevent blood clotting and maintain blood flow

A deficiency in erythropoietin will result in anemia. The deficiency may result from kidney disease where erythropoietin secretion is compromised, or it may have a genetic origin.

Diagnosis of Erythropoietin Deficiency Anemia:

An anemia secondary to decreased EPO can be diagnosed by:

- Blood levels showing low EPO levels
- A complete blood count (CBC) to help differentiate EPO deficiency from other causes of anemia
- Renal function tests (e.g., BUN, serum creatinine, estimated glomerular filtration rate) to determine if the decreased erythropoietin is due to renal disease
- Bone marrow evaluation (to detect an abnormality or deficiency in erythropoiesis)

Treatment of EPO Deficiency:

- Manage the underlying cause (e.g., kidney dysfunction).
- Administer EPO or other erythropoiesis-stimulating agents to stimulate RBC production.
- Blood transfusion
- Nutritional support (adequate iron, B vitamins, protein, and other nutrients important in red cell production)

Chapter 13 **Stomach and Intestines**

While the stomach and intestines do not have specialized endocrine glands, they do produce and release quite a few hormones that play a role in regulating digestion. These include:

- Peptide YY
- Gastrin
- Serotonin
- Cholecystokinin
- Secretin
- Gastric-Inhibitory Peptide
- Motilin
- Ghrelin
- Glucagon-Like Peptide-1 (GLP-1)

Peptide YY (PYY)

PYY is a hormone produced by specialized cells in the lining of the ileum and colon. It is released in response to food intake and slows the transit of blood through the gut. PYY acts on the brain to decrease appetite and reduce eating.

Gastrin

Gastrin, produced by G cells in the stomach, binds to receptors on the surface of the acid-producing parietal cells in the stomach lining and stimulates gastric acid secretion; it also increases gastric motility. Gastrin release is stimulated by:

- The presence of food in the stomach, which stretches the stomach wall
- Certain amino acids (particularly phenylalanine and tryptophan)
- Vagal nerve stimulation

Excess gastrin can lead to gastroesophageal reflux disease (GERD) or peptic ulcers. In **Zollinger-Ellison syndrome**, a gastrinoma (which can be benign or malignant), usually in the pancreas or duodenum, secretes excess amount of gastrin. The syndrome is marked by peptic ulcers, diarrhea, weight loss, and sometimes GI bleeding and perforation. Gastrinomas can occur sporadically or as part of the inherited condition **Multiple Endocrine Neoplasia type 1 (MEN1)**.

Excess gastrin can have several causes:

- Zollinger-Ellison syndrome or neuroendocrine tumors that secrete gastrin
- Chronic atrophic gastritis. Inflammation and degradation of the stomach lining can stimulate the G cells to produce more gastrin to compensate.
- Hypercalcemia can stimulate gastrin release.
- Helicobacter pylori infections in its initial inflammatory stage
- Antral G-cell hyperplasia, where there is an excess number of gastrin-producing cells in the stomach antrum
- Kidney failure may result in decreased clearance of gastrin, leading to increased gastrin levels.

- Medications that decrease stomach acid, such as proton pump inhibitors and H2 receptor antagonists, can, by decreasing the acidity, lead to feedback that stimulates more gastrin release. Increased gastrin can also result after a partial gastrectomy.
- Stress can lead to increased gastrin levels.
- Autoimmune gastritis damages gastric parietal cells. The reduced acid triggers a feedback action that increases gastrin.

Clues to the diagnosis of Zollinger-Ellison syndrome include:

- Elevated gastrin levels along with high gastric acidity (low pH)
- CT scan and MRI can help identify tumors in the pancreas or duodenal wall, as can endoscopic ultrasound. Somatostatin receptor scintigraphy (*octreotide scan*) can help locate tumors that express somatostatin receptors, including gastrinomas.
- In one type of **gastrin stimulation test**, the patient is administered secretin, which normally inhibits the release of gastrin. Significantly *elevated* levels of gastrin after the test may suggest a gastrinoma, in which gastrin secretion is paradoxically increased by secretin due to abnormal secretin receptors. Other conditions with high gastrin, like atrophic gastritis, do not exhibit an increase in gastrin levels using the same test (**Fig. 13-1**).

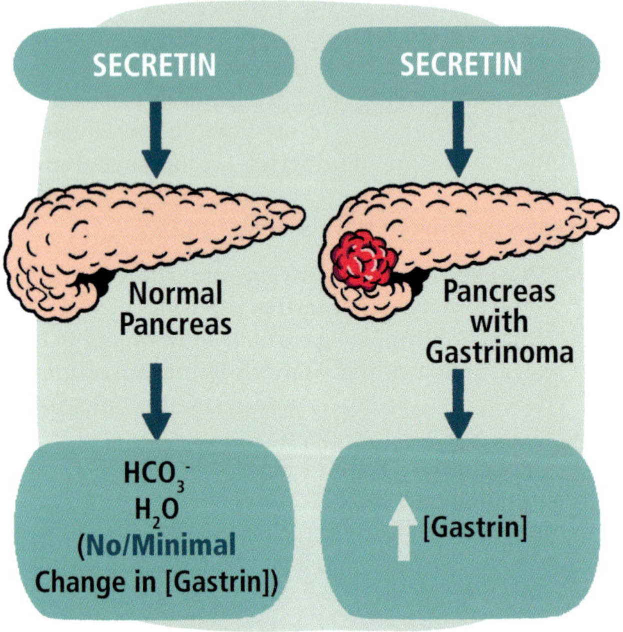

Fig. 13-1. Secretin test.

The treatment for gastrin excess includes:

- Proton pump inhibitors
- Surgery for gastrinoma. This may include partial or total gastrectomy.
- Medications targeting gastrinomas (e.g., somatostatin analogs, chemotherapy)
- Management of complications (peptic ulcer, GI bleed)

Pernicious Anemia

Pernicious anemia is caused by the body's inability to absorb vitamin B12 from the gastrointestinal tract, typically due to a lack of *intrinsic factor*. Intrinsic factor is a protein produced by parietal cells in the stomach lining; it binds to vitamin B12 to facilitate its absorption in the small intestine. The most common reason for the lack of intrinsic factor is an autoimmune response against intrinsic factor or against the parietal cells, leading to their destruction or dysfunction. This autoimmune condition often results in *atrophic gastritis*, a thinning of the stomach lining, which further reduces the production of intrinsic factor and stomach acid necessary for B12 absorption. Without enough vitamin B12, the body cannot produce enough healthy red blood cells, leading to anemia and a range of neurological symptoms. The loss of stomach acid triggers an increase in gastrin, which tries to stimulate the remaining parietal cells to work harder.

B12 deficiency can be diagnosed by the combination of characteristic hematologic findings, low serum B12 levels, antibodies to intrinsic factor, high gastrin levels with *reduced* stomach acidity (high pH), and the neurologic exam, which may show gait and other abnormalities.

The treatment for B12 deficiency is B12, given orally, or when malabsorption is at the root of the problem, by intramuscular injections of B12.

Serotonin

Serotonin (5-hydroxytryptamine, or 5-HT) is a neurotransmitter and hormone that is found in high concentrations in the stomach and small intestine (about 90-95% of the body's serotonin is found in the intestines). It stimulates gut motility and decreases appetite.

Excess serotonin can be pathological:

- **Serotonin syndrome**: This occurs when there is too much serotonin in the brain. There are changes in mental status (anxiety, confusion), autonomic hyperactivity (hyperthermia, flushing, tachycardia, hypertension, tachypnea), neuromuscular problems (tremors, muscle rigidity, incoordination), and more severe symptoms in some (rhabdomyolysis, seizures, unconsciousness). Serotonin syndrome is usually associated with the use of certain medications, e.g., selective serotonin reuptake inhibitors (SSRIs), tricyclic antidepressants, and certain anti-migraine medications, and monoamine oxidase inhibitors (MAOIs). (MAOIs inhibit the activity of monoamine oxidase, an enzyme that breaks down serotonin, norepinephrine, and dopamine, so MAOIs cause the levels of these neurotransmitters to increase.)

  There are no specific lab tests to diagnose serotonin syndrome. Diagnosis is more an exclusion of other possible causes of the patient's symptoms.

- **Carcinoid syndrome**: Certain tumors produce excessive serotonin. Carcinoid tumors can secrete other substances as well, such as histamine and gastrin, leading to symptoms of flushing, diarrhea, wheezing and other symptoms.
- Certain types of **autism** may involve elevated levels of serotonin.

The treatment of excess serotonin includes discontinuing serotonergic drugs, administering anti-serotonergic medication (e.g., *cyproheptadine*), and management of symptoms.

Cholecystokinin (CCK)

CCK is primarily produced by specialized cells in the duodenum and jejunum. It is released in response to fats and proteins in the small intestine. CCK stimulates the release of digestive enzymes from the pancreas, promotes the contraction of the gallbladder to release bile, and reduces appetite.

Secretin

Secretin, produced in the duodenum, plays a role in regulating the pH balance in the small intestine. It is released in response to the presence of acidic chyme (partially digested food) that enters the small intestine from the stomach. Secretin reduces gastrin secretion and stimulates the pancreas to release bicarbonate-rich pancreatic juice, which helps neutralize the acidic chyme.

Gastric Inhibitory Peptide (GIP)

GIP, also known as glucose-dependent insulinotropic peptide, is produced by cells in the duodenum and jejunum. It is released in response to the presence of nutrients, particularly glucose and fatty acids. GIP stimulates the release of insulin from the pancreas, promotes glucose uptake and utilization by cells, and inhibits gastric acid secretion.

Motilin

Motilin is produced in the duodenum and jejunum. It stimulates the contraction of smooth muscles in the stomach and small intestine, helping to propel food through the digestive system.

Ghrelin

Ghrelin (the "hunger hormone"), is mainly produced in the stomach. It stimulates hunger and increases food intake. Its levels rise before meals and drop after eating, telling us when it's time to stop eating. It also stimulates gastric emptying and promotes fat storage, putting away energy for future needs. Ghrelin also stimulates the release of growth hormone from the anterior pituitary gland.

Glucagon-Like Peptide-1 (GLP-1)

GLP-1 is one of a group of GI hormones called **incretins** that can enhance the secretion of insulin and suppress the secretion of glucagon from the pancreas when glucose is elevated. It also suppresses gastric emptying and induces satiety. (Although GLP-1 is called "glucagon-like," that is only in terms of structure, as it has an effect opposite that of glucagon. While glucagon raises blood sugar, GLP-1 enhances insulin secretion.) GLP-1 receptor agonists, e.g., *exanatide, liraglutide, lixisenatide, dulaglutide, semaglutide (Ozempic)*, are used in the treatment of type 2 diabetes, as they decrease glucose and help weight loss. **DPP-4 inhibitors**, e.g., *sitagliptin, saxagliptin, linagliptin, alogliptin*, inhibit the enzyme DPP-4, which normally breaks down native GLP-1. DPP-4 inhibitors are used mainly for the treatment of type 2 diabetes.

Chapter 14 **Placenta**

The placenta is critical during pregnancy for exchanging nutrients and waste between mother and fetus. It forms shortly after the fertilized egg implants into the uterine wall, usually around 6-10 days after ovulation. The placenta produces several hormones that are important in maintaining the pregnancy and supporting fetal development:

- **Human Chorionic Gonadotropin (hCG)**
- **Relaxin**
- **Human Placental Lactogen (hPL)**

Human Chorionic Gonadotropin (hCG)

hCG stimulates the corpus luteum to produce progesterone in early pregnancy to help maintain the fetus and the health of the uterine endometrial lining. hCG also stimulates the mammary glands to grow, as part of the body's preparation for breastfeeding. By the end of the first trimester (about 10-12 weeks), hCG ensures that the placenta continues to develop and take over the role of producing progesterone and estrogen. Progesterone supports the continuing growth of the placenta and fetus, maintains the uterine lining, and suppresses premature uterine contractions.

hCG is the earliest detectable indicator of pregnancy; its production starts after implantation (not after fertilization), which generally occurs about 6-10 days after ovulation. Blood pregnancy tests for hCG can detect pregnancy earlier than urine tests, sometimes as early as 6-8 days after ovulation.

Over-the-counter urine pregnancy tests for hCG are generally accurate and can often detect pregnancy as early as the first day of a missed menstrual period although some tests claim to detect hCG even a few days before the missed period. Tests taken too early may not yield accurate results because the hCG levels may still be too low for detection. For the most accurate results, it is often recommended to take the test one week after the missed period. If a negative result is obtained but pregnancy is still suspected, the test should be repeated after a few days to a week.

Excess hCG production may occur with rare tumors (hydatiform moles, choriocarcinoma, placental tumors, molar pregnancy [a tumor of the uterus from a nonviable pregnancy], testicular, ovarian, and other cancers), or an ectopic pregnancy. Signs may include irregular or absent menstrual periods, breast tenderness, enlarged ovaries, nausea and vomiting, or abdominal pain. Tumors may be detected in imaging studies, and, depending on the type, may require surgery, radiation, or chemotherapy.

Relaxin

Relaxin relaxes and softens various connective tissues during pregnancy, including ligaments and the cervix, to facilitate childbirth and accommodate fetal growth.

Human Placental Lactogen (hPL)

Human Placental Lactogen contributes to breast changes during pregnancy, including increased sensitivity to prolactin. It increases the breakdown of fats to provide free fatty acid energy for the mother, and contributes to increased insulin resistance in the mother, ensuring more glucose for the fetus.

Sometimes the excess glucose from insulin resistance is manifest as gestational diabetes. This can result in:

- *Fetal macrosomia.* (High birth weight – excess glucose stimulates the fetal pancreas to produce more insulin; insulin promotes storage of triglycerides in adipose tissue.)
- *Polyhydramnios* (excess amniotic fluid) due to increased fetal urine production as the baby tries to get rid of the excess glucose it's receiving when the mother has diabetes
- *Hypoglycemia in the newborn.* (High insulin produced by the fetus to deal with the high glucose persists after birth when the mother is no longer supplying glucose.) Low glucose in the newborn needs to be monitored and carefully managed. Children born to mothers with gestational diabetes are at a higher risk for obesity and type 2 diabetes, which need to be considered in their postnatal care and follow-up.

Chapter 15 **Adipose Tissue**

Leptin (Fig. 15-1)

Leptin (often referred to as the "satiety hormone") is primarily produced by adipose (fat) tissue. It plays an important role in regulating appetite, energy balance, and metabolism:

- **Regulation of appetite:** Leptin acts on the hypothalamus to reduce appetite and increase feelings of fullness, helping to regulate eating. Leptin levels increase with increased body fat, which helps control food intake. However, in some cases of obesity, *leptin resistance* may occur, where the body becomes less responsive to the signals of leptin, leading to overeating and weight gain.
- **Energy expenditure and metabolism**: When leptin levels are elevated, it signals to the brain that energy stores are sufficient, leading to an increase in metabolic rate and energy expenditure. This helps prevent excessive weight gain. Leptin stimulates the hypothalamus to secrete thyrotropin-releasing hormone (TRH). TRH stimulates the pituitary gland to secrete thyroid-stimulating hormone (THS). TSH stimulates the thyroid gland to synthesize and release thyroid hormones (T3 and T4), which increase metabolic rate.
- **Regulation of reproductive function:** Leptin facilitates pituitary gonadotropin secretion. Increased body fat energy reserves and elevated leptin levels are associated with early onset puberty. Low levels of leptin and body fat, as seen in starvation, can lead to amenorrhea and delayed puberty. In an evolutionary sense, leptin helps ensure that reproduction happens under favorable conditions, where there is enough food and energy.
- **Immune system regulation:** Leptin also activates certain components of the immune system. This may be a reason why obesity is often linked to a state of chronic low-grade-inflammation and susceptibility to certain diseases.
- **Other functions**: Leptin can increase insulin sensitivity, promoting glucose uptake in peripheral tissues and lowering blood glucose levels. Reducing food intake can also reduce glucose. Leptin may decrease insulin secretion in response to the decrease in glucose. It can also promote bone formation by stimulating the differentiation of osteoblasts (which form bone) and inhibiting the formation and function of osteoclasts (which break down bone).

Adinopectin

Adiponectin is a hormone secreted by fat cells. It has insulin-enhancing and anti-inflammatory effects.

Obese individuals generally have *lower* adiponectin levels than lean individuals (unlike leptins, which tend to be higher in obese individuals).

Insulin sensitivity: Adiponectin helps the body respond better to insulin's actions, resulting in more efficient glucose uptake by cells. In obesity, adiponectin

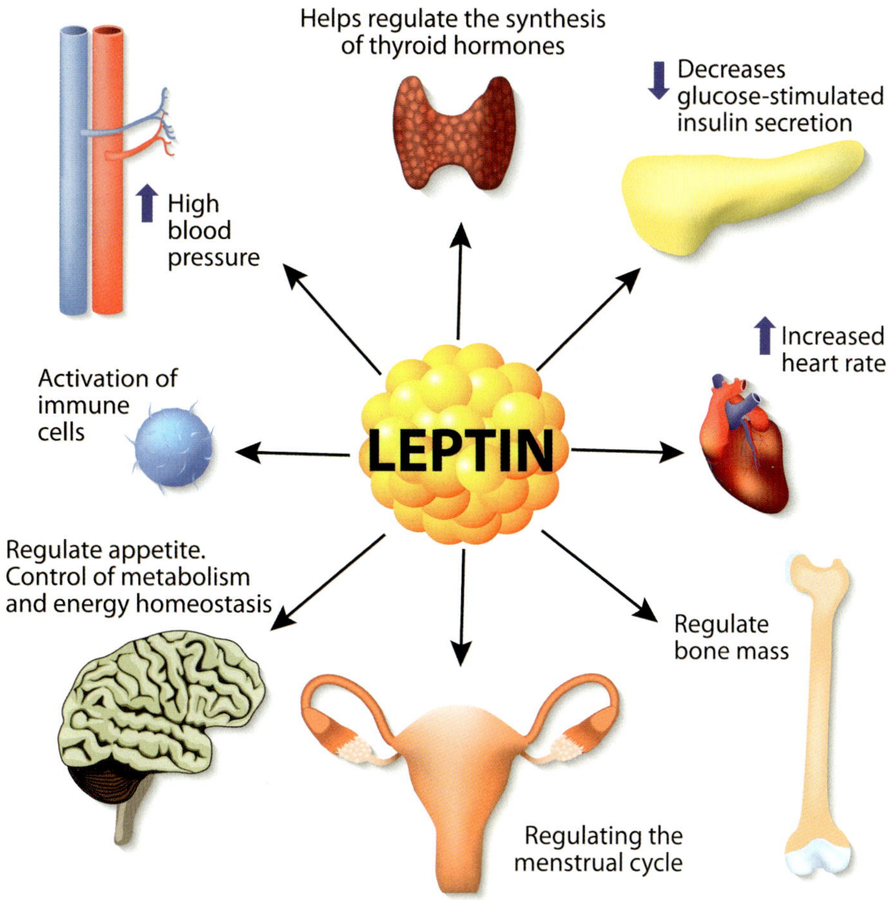

Fig. 15-1. Functions of leptin.

levels decline, contributing to decreased insulin sensitivity, which can lead to insulin resistance and an increased risk of type 2 diabetes.

Anti-inflammatory properties: Adiponectin helps to suppress inflammation, partly by reducing the production of inflammatory cytokines. Lower adiponectin levels in obesity may contribute to a pro-inflammatory state, which is associated with various obesity-related complications, such as cardiovascular disease.

People with excess visceral fat (fat around internal organs) tend to have lower adiponectin levels compared to those where the excess fat is subcutaneous (fat under the skin). Visceral fat is associated with a higher risk of metabolic disorders, such as insulin-resistant type 2 diabetes, metabolic syndrome, cardiovascular diseases, dyslipidemia, and non-alcoholic fatty liver disease. Some studies have shown an association between visceral obesity and an increased risk of developing certain cancers, such as colorectal and pancreatic cancer.

Weight loss has been shown to increase adiponectin levels in individuals with obesity. This is one of the positive effects of weight loss, as higher adiponectin levels are associated with improved metabolic health.

Genetic variations can influence adiponectin levels. Some people may have genetic predispositions that lead to lower adiponectin production, making them more susceptible to obesity-related metabolic disturbances.

Hormones That Decrease Appetite

Hormones that *decrease* appetite include:

- **Leptin**: Produced by fat cells, leptin signals the hypothalamus to reduce appetite (see above discussion).
- **Peptide YY:** Released by cells in the small intestine and colon, peptide YY is secreted after eating and reduces appetite by signaling the brain and slowing gastric emptying.
- **Glucagon-like peptide-1 (GLP-1)**: Secreted by the small intestine in response to eating, GLP-1

contributes to feelings of fullness by signaling the hypothalamus, which decreases appetite. It also slows down gastric motility and emptying, prolonging the feeling of fullness (**Fig. 15-2**). In addition, it enhances the secretion of insulin and reduces the action of glucagon, which is a reason that GLP-1 agonists (e.g., *liraglutide, exenatide,* and *dulaglutide*) are used in treating type 2 diabetes – for glucose control and weight loss.

- **Oxyntomodulin**, co-secreted with GLP-1 and PYY from the GI tract, helps to reduce food intake by slowing gastric emptying and signaling the brain, resulting in a feeling of satiety. It also stimulates insulin secretion and inhibits glucagon secretion.
- **Cholecystokinin**, produced in the duodenum in response to the presence of food in the stomach and small intestine, acts on receptors in the brain to induce feelings of fullness and satiety.
- **Insulin** can contribute to feelings of satiety by promoting nutrient uptake and storage in cells, which could lead to a temporary decrease in the need for food intake. (Cortisol, while not technically considered a "hunger hormone," can *increase* appetite by counteracting insulin, particularly in times of stress.)
- **Amylin**, co-released with insulin by the pancreas, suppresses glucagon and reduces blood sugar. It also slows gastric emptying, promoting feelings of fullness. It signals the brainstem and hypothalamus to reduce feelings of hunger and promote a sense of fullness.

Hormones That Increase Appetite

Ghrelin, often called the "hunger hormone," is primarily produced in the stomach and released when the stomach is empty. It signals the brain to be hungry and eat. Typically, ghrelin levels rise before a meal, stimulating hunger, and fall shortly afterward.

Neuropeptide Y (NPY), produced in the hypothalamus, stimulates eating and is influenced by factors like stress and fasting.

Agouti-related protein (AgRP), released in the hypothalamus, acts as an antagonist to melanocortin receptors, promoting food intake. (Melanocortins are derivatives of the same protein that cleaves to form ACTH and melanocyte-stimulating hormone.) The melanocortin alpha-MSH, produced in the hypothalamus, promotes feelings of fullness and can lead to reduced food intake. AgRP, by antagonizing melanocortin receptors, increases appetite.

Orexin (hypocretin), produced in the hypothalamus, promotes wakefulness and stimulates appetite.

Other than hormones, there are psychological factors that increase appetite. Emotions – boredom, sadness, and other emotional states – can trigger "emotional eating." Simply seeing or smelling food can trigger the desire to eat, a la Pavlov.

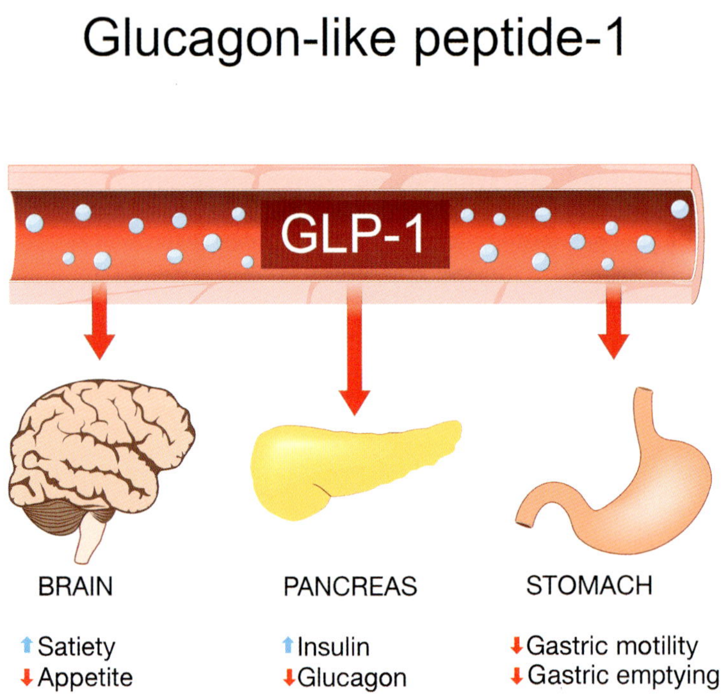

Fig. 15-2. Functions of GLP-1.

Chapter 16 **Multiple Endocrine Neoplasia**

Multiple Endocrine Neoplasia (MEN) is a group of rare autosomal dominant genetic disorders that affect the endocrine system. MEN is characterized by the development of tumors in multiple endocrine glands, typically involving two or more glands.

MEN1, MEN2A, and MEN2B

There are three main types of MEN:

1. **Multiple Endocrine Neoplasia type 1 (MEN1)**: MEN1 is caused by mutations in the MEN1 gene. It is characterized by an increased risk of developing tumors of the **parathyroid glands** (hyperparathyroidism), **pancreas** (e.g., an insulinoma or gastrinoma) and **pituitary gland** (e.g., a prolactinoma or a growth hormone-secreting tumor) and which may start to function at different times and degrees.
2. **Multiple Endocrine Neoplasia type 2A (MEN2A)**: MEN2A is caused by mutations in the RET proto-oncogene. It is characterized by the development of tumors in the **thyroid gland** (medullary thyroid carcinoma), **adrenal glands** (pheochromocytoma), and **parathyroid glands** (primary hyperparathyroidism).
3. **Multiple Endocrine Neoplasia type 2B (MEN2B)**: MEN2B is also caused by mutations in the RET proto-oncogene. It, too, is characterized by the development of tumors in the **thyroid gland** (aggressive medullary thyroid carcinoma) and **adrenal glands** (pheochromocytoma), as well as benign mucosal tumors that may appear on the lips, tongue, inner side of the cheeks, eyelids and conjunctiva. Individuals with MEN2B may also exhibit distinctive physical features, such as a marfanoid body habitus and ganglioneuromas (which are benign and non-functioning) of the gastrointestinal tract. MEN2B does not typically involve the parathyroid glands.

The tumors associated with MEN can be benign or malignant.

Diagnosis of MEN

Diagnosis involves assessing hormone levels, genetic testing to identify the specific gene mutation and medical imaging to detect and monitor the presence of tumors.

Treatment of MEN

Treatment options depend on the type and location of tumors and may include surgery, radiation, medication, or other targeted therapies. For instance, in MEN1, calcimimetics (e.g., *cinacalcet*) may be prescribed to decrease PTH secretion in hyperparathyroidism; *tyrosine kinase inhibitors* (e.g., *vandetanib, cabozantinib*) can inhibit cell growth and division in medullary thyroid cancer. Symptomatic medication can alleviate the symptoms of pheochromocytoma such as hypertension and tachycardia.

It's important for individuals with MEN and their families to undergo regular medical screenings and genetic counseling to manage the condition and assess the risk of passing it on to future generations. Although MEN is rare, the MEN syndromes are autosomal dominant, which means that each child of an affected individual has a 50% chance of inheriting the dominant gene.

Neuroendocrine Tumors

The MEN tumor syndromes should be distinguished from **neuroendocrine tumors (NETs)**. Neuroendocrine cells are cells that can receive nerve signals and release hormones in response. These kinds of cells are scattered throughout the body, in the GI tract, lungs, pancreas, adrenal medulla, thyroid, pituitary gland, pineal gland, hypothalamus, skin, prostate, and reproductive organs. They play a role in translating neural signals into endocrine responses in their respective organs. NET tumors can be benign or malignant, secretory or non-secretory. The secretory ones include *insulinomas, gastrinomas*, and *carcinoid tumors*.

Carcinoid tumors can produce vasoactive substances (such as serotonin, histamine, tachykinins, and prostaglandins), which can lead to *carcinoid syndrome*, marked by flushing, diarrhea, bronchoconstriction, and eventually, carcinoid heart disease, which affects the heart valves and can lead to right-sided heart failure. The syndrome usually arises when the tumors metastasize to the liver; the liver usually metabolizes and inactivates the substances secreted by these tumors, but when there are liver metastases, the substances can bypass the liver's filtering mechanism and enter the general circulation, causing symptoms. Over time, this can lead to fibrosis of heart valves especially on the right side, leading to tricuspid valve insufficiency or pulmonary valve stenosis.

Diagnosis of Neuroendocrine Tumors

- Clinical assessment of symptoms and physical exam
- Laboratory tests:
  - Hormonal assays, e.g., 5-HIAA, a serotonin metabolite, in the urine for suspected carcinoid tumors
  - *Chromogranin A and B*. These are neurosecretory proteins that can be detected in the blood as general markers for NETs.
  - Routine blood tests for liver and kidney function, CBC, etc. to assess general health
- Imaging studies:
  - CT or MRI, ultrasound, chest X-ray or bone scan to visualize tumors
  - Octreoscan (uses a radiolabeled somatostatin analog to detect tumors with somatostatin receptors)
  - PET scan (uses different tracers like 68Ga-Dotatate or FDG to help detect NETs and their metastases)
- Biopsy
- Cardiac echocardiography
- Genetic testing (most NETs do not have a known genetic cause)

Treatment of Neuroendocrine Tumors

- Surgery to remove or debulk the tumor
- Somatostatin analogs (e.g., *octreotide* or *lanreotide*) mimic somatostatin and decrease secretion of various hormones.
- Peptide receptor radionuclide therapy uses a radioactive molecule combined with a drug that targets specific receptors on the tumor cells (e.g., lutetium Lu177-Dotatate).
- Chemotherapy. Targeted therapies target specific molecular pathways involved in tumor growth, e.g., *everolimus, sunitinib*.
- Hepatic artery embolization (blocks blood supply to the tumor metastases)
- Radiation
- Supportive care

Autoimmune Polyendocrine Syndromes

Autoimmune polyendocrine syndromes (APS) are a group of rare autoimmune disorders which, unlike the oversecreting MEN and neuroendocrine tumors, are characterized by the simultaneous or sequential destruction of function in multiple endocrine glands. These syndromes include:

- **Autoimmune polyendocrine syndrome type 1 (APS-1)**, also known as **autoimmune polyendocrinopathy-candidiasis-ectodermal dystrophy (APECED)**. APS-1 is a rare genetic disorder characterized by the dysfunction of multiple endocrine organs. It typically manifests in childhood or adolescence and is caused by mutations in the AIRE (Autoimmune Regulator) gene. The affected glands may include the *parathyroid glands, adrenal glands*, and *pancreatic islets*, leading to hypoparathyroidism, adrenal insufficiency, and diabetes.

- **Autoimmune polyendocrine syndrome type 2 (APS-2)**: APS-2 is more common than APS-1 and usually develops in adulthood. It is characterized by the presence of autoimmune Addison's disease (*adrenal insufficiency*) in combination with another endocrine disorder, such as autoimmune thyroid disease (Hashimoto's thyroiditis or Graves' disease) or type 1 diabetes. APS-2 is associated with certain genetic predispositions, such as specific human leukocyte antigen (HLA) alleles.
- **Autoimmune polyendocrine syndrome type 3 (APS-3)**: Resembles APS-2, but without Addison's disease.
- **Other polyendocrine syndromes**: There are additional rare autoimmune polyendocrine syndromes with different combinations of affected endocrine glands.

Diagnosis of Autoimmune Polyendocrine Syndromes

- Look for the presence of multiple endocrine dysfunctions.
- Assess autoantibody profiles.
- Conduct genetic testing if applicable.
- Consider clinical criteria specific to each subtype.

Treatment of Autoimmune Polyendocrine Syndromes

Treatment primarily focuses on managing the particular endocrine disorders, such as hormone replacement therapy for adrenal insufficiency, thyroid hormone replacement for thyroid disease, blood sugar management for diabetes, and immune suppressors for the autoimmune component, as well as symptomatic management (e.g., calcium and vitamin D supplementation for hypoparathyroidism). Regular medical monitoring and surveillance are essential to detect and manage any additional endocrine dysfunctions or complications associated with APS.

Chapter 17 **Disorders of Sexual Development (DSD)**

A person's sex assigned at birth typically refers to the classification as male or female based on physical attributes, such as chromosomes, hormone levels, and reproductive anatomy. Disruption of mechanisms in these areas can lead to congenital disorders of sexual development (DSD). DSD is a physical issue that should be distinguished from the term "gender dysphoria" which refers to discomfort a person may have about a mismatch between their preferred gender identity and their sex assigned at birth.

Genetic Disorders

Disorders of sexual development (DSD) can have different causes, some involving genetic mutations or an abnormal number of chromosomes, leading to deficient hormonal or structural attributes. Examples include:

- **Hypogonadism**: Hypogonadism is a condition in which the testes or ovaries produce insufficient amounts of sex hormones, particularly testosterone in males and estrogen/progesterone in females.

There are two main types of hypogonadism:

Primary hypogonadism occurs when the testes or ovaries are unable to produce enough sex hormones due to intrinsic dysfunction. It can be caused by genetic disorders, autoimmune conditions, chemo- or radiation therapy, infections, certain medications, or testicular or ovarian injury. In primary hypogonadism, the levels of follicle-stimulating hormone (FSH) and luteinizing hormone (LH) in the blood are typically *elevated* as the body tries to stimulate the gonads to produce hormones. Hence the name *hypergonadotropic hypogonadism.*

Secondary hypogonadism (also known as *hypogonadotropic hypogonadism*) occurs when there is an inadequacy in the hypothalamus or pituitary gland that interferes with the production of FSH and LH. As a result, the gonads receive insufficient stimulation to produce sex hormones. Secondary hypogonadism can be caused by conditions such as tumors, infections, head trauma, genetic disorders, or certain medications. In secondary hypogonadism, the levels of FSH and LH are generally *low*.

Depending on the age of onset and degree of hormonal deficiency, and whether it affects males or females, it can lead to anatomical abnormalities at birth (e.g., micropenis, undescended testes, ambiguous genitalia), or delayed or absent puberty with lack of development of secondary sexual characteristics.

- **Turner Syndrome** (45,X) is a genetic disorder that affects females, characterized by the absence or abnormality of one of the X chromosomes. It results in a range of physical and developmental abnormalities, including short stature, delayed puberty, infertility, webbed neck, and certain heart and kidney defects. It is a form of hypogonadism with insufficient production of sex hormones, including estrogen, and primary ovarian insufficiency.

- **Klinefelter Syndrome** (47,XXY) is a chromosomal disorder that affects males, usually resulting from an extra X chromosome (XXY). It leads to underdeveloped testes, low testosterone levels, delayed or incomplete puberty, and infertility; it may cause physical and cognitive symptoms such as tall stature, gynecomastia (breast enlargement), and learning difficulties.
- **Swyer Syndrome** (46,XY Gonadal Dysgenesis) is a form of gonadal dysgenesis that affects individuals with a Y chromosome (typically associated with male development) but with abnormal or absent testes, female external genitalia and usually a uterus and fallopian tubes, but who lack functional ovaries. Individuals with Swyer syndrome are typically assigned female at birth.
- **Androgen Insensitivity Syndrome** (AIS; Testicular Feminization Syndrome) is a genetic condition in which individuals with male sex chromosomes (XY) are partially or completely insensitive to androgens. This results in incomplete or absent development of male sexual characteristics. Depending on the degree of androgen insensitivity, individuals with AIS may have female or ambiguous external genitalia.
- **Congenital Adrenal Hyperplasia** (CAH) is a group of genetic disorders that have a defect in one of the enzymatic pathways of adrenal gland synthesis of cortisol, aldosterone, and/or androgens (see **Fig. 5-9**):
  - *21-hydroxylase deficiency* (the most common): Reduced cortisol and aldosterone, and increased androgens, causing ambiguous genitalia in females, early virilization in both males and females, and infertility.
  - *11 beta-hydroxylase deficiency*: Reduced cortisol and increased androgens and deoxy-corticosterone, with virilization and hypertension.
  - *17 alpha-hydroxylase deficiency*: Reduced cortisol and sex steroids, and increased mineralocorticoids, with hypertension, hypokalemia, and sexual infantilism.
  - *3 beta-hydroxysteroid dehydrogenase deficiency*: Decreased cortisol, aldosterone, and androgens, with *undervirilization* in males (decreased testosterone), and *virilization* in females (decreased estrogens with accumulation of DHEA, which can be converted to some testosterone by alternative pathways).
  - *Aromatase deficiency*: Impaired conversion of testosterone to estrogen results in accumulation of androgens, with masculinization and infertility in females and impaired bone mineralization in both males and females due to the lack of estrogen.
  - *P450scc deficiency*: Impaired conversion of cholesterol to pregnenolone (the rate-limiting step in adrenal hormone production) decreases the production of all the adrenal cortical hormones.
- **Premature Ovarian Insufficiency** (POI), also known as *premature menopause* or *early ovarian failure*, occurs when the ovaries stop functioning normally before the age of 40. It results in a decline in estrogen production, leading to irregular or absent menstrual periods, infertility, and menopausal symptoms.
- **Mixed Gonadal Dysgenesis** is atypical gonadal development involving both testicular and ovarian tissue. The individual may have external genitalia that are ambiguous or resemble female anatomy, and gonads may be a mix of testicular and ovarian tissue.
- **Hermaphroditism**, also known as **intersex**, is a condition where an individual is born with reproductive or sexual anatomy that does not fit typical definitions of male or female. The causes of hermaphroditism can be complex and multifactorial, involving genetic, hormonal, and environmental factors.

  True hermaphroditism (ovotesticular DSD) is a rare condition where an individual has both ovarian and testicular tissues. This can result in the presence of both male and female reproductive organs. True hermaphroditism is often associated with chromosomal variations, such as having both XX and XY chromosomes in the same individual (*chimerism* or *mosaicism*).

  Pseudohermaphroditism refers to individuals who have ambiguous genitalia that may appear either male or female, but the internal reproductive organs may not correspond to the external appearance. Pseudohermaphroditism can be further categorized into *male pseudohermaphroditism* and *female pseudohermaphroditism*, depending on the presence of testes or ovaries, respectively. Certain kinds of hermaphroditism can run in families.

  It is important to note that being intersex is a naturally occurring variation in humans, and while some would categorize it as a disorder, others do not. Historically, medical professionals often recommended surgeries or other medical interventions for intersex babies to make their physical appearance conform to male or female norms. However, this approach has been the subject of significant controversy, as these interventions can have lifelong consequences and were often done without the informed consent of the intersex individual. Many advocates and medical professionals now promote a more patient-centered approach that involves the individual (and their family, if the person is a minor) in the decision-making process.

Diagnosis of DSD

Diagnosis may involve a combination of:

- Medical/family history and physical examination
- Chromosome analysis (karyotype) and gene sequencing to identify specific mutations and chromosome anomalies
- Hormone testing, e.g., FSH, LH, estradiol, testosterone, prolactin (elevated levels of prolactin can suppress gonadotropin production and lead to hypogonadism), and, in some cases, anti-Müllerian hormone (which has important functions in the regulation of the female and male reproductive system)
- Imaging studies to assess the structure and function of the hypothalamus, pituitary gland, testes, or ovaries. This may include magnetic resonance imaging (MRI), computed tomography (CT), or ultrasound.

Treatment of DSD

- **A multidisciplinary approach** with a team of pediatric endocrinologists, pediatric surgeons, psychologists, geneticists, and social workers may help ensure comprehensive and holistic care.
- **Individualized decision-making**: Treatment decisions should involve the informed consent of the individual (when appropriate) and their parents or guardians, taking into account the individual's physical, psychological, and social needs. Discussions should focus on the available treatment options, potential benefits, risks, and long-term implications.
- **Hormone therapy** may be used (testosterone in males; estrogen and progesterone in females) to help promote appropriate sexual development and secondary sexual characteristics. Hormones can be used either to suppress or stimulate the development of specific characteristics based on the individual's specific condition and goals.
- **Medication adjustments**: Certain medications can cause hypogonadism, whether by directly affecting the gonads (primary hypogonadism) or acting on the hypothalamus or pituitary gland (secondary or central hypogonadism). Chemotherapy drugs can damage the gonads. Opioids, chronic use of glucocorticoids, and other medications can affect the hypothalamus/pituitary axis. Adjusting or discontinuing the medication may be necessary.
- **Surgical interventions** may be considered to correct anatomical anomalies or align the physical appearance of the genitalia with the individual's gender identity, improve urinary or reproductive function, or address specific medical needs, based on the individual's specific circumstances.
- **Long-term follow-up**: Regular monitoring and long-term follow-up with the healthcare team are important to assess the individual's physical and psychological well-being, monitor hormone levels, address any complications or concerns, and adjust treatment plans as needed.

Disorders of Puberty

Puberty may be delayed or premature.

Delayed puberty refers to a delay or absence of the physical and hormonal changes that typically occur during adolescence. In girls, puberty is considered delayed if there is no breast development by age 13 and no menstruation (menarche) by age 16 or within 5 years of the onset of breast development. In boys, puberty is considered delayed if there is no testicular enlargement by age 14 and more than 5 years pass between the first appearance of testicular enlargement and the completion of genital growth.

Premature puberty is usually defined as the onset of secondary sexual characteristics before 8 years of age in girls and 9 years in boys.

Delayed Puberty

Delayed puberty can have various causes, including:

1. **Constitutional Delay**: This is the most common cause. It occurs when there is a natural variation in the timing of puberty, a delay in the activation of the hypothalamic-pituitary-gonadal axis. Children with constitutional delay often have a family history of late puberty, and they eventually go through puberty but at a later age than their peers.
2. **Chronic Illness**: Certain chronic medical conditions, such as cystic fibrosis, kidney disease, malnutrition, and celiac disease, can affect the hormonal balance and delay the onset of puberty.

3. **Hormonal Disorders**: Disorders affecting the production or function of hormones involved in puberty can cause delayed puberty, e.g., hypothyroidism (thyroid hormone is important for normal growth and development), hypogonadism (impaired function of the gonads), and conditions affecting the pituitary gland or hypothalamus, such as a primary hormonal deficiency or physical damage (e.g., compression by a craniopharygioma).
4. **Genetic or Chromosomal Disorders**: Certain genetic or chromosomal abnormalities, such as Klinefelter syndrome (XXY), Turner syndrome (XO), and other conditions, can be associated with delayed puberty.
5. **Primary Ovarian Insufficiency (POI)**: Also known as premature ovarian failure, POI occurs when the ovaries stop functioning before the age of 40. It can cause delayed or absent puberty in affected individuals.
6. **Structural Abnormalities**: Structural abnormalities of the reproductive system, such as congenital absence of the uterus or vagina, can lead to delayed puberty.
7. **Medications**: Certain medications, such as some chemotherapy drugs and medications used to treat chronic conditions, e.g., chronic corticosteroid use, and some anti-epileptic and anti-psychotic drugs can affect hormone production and delay puberty.
8. **Environmental Toxins**: Some plastics, pesticides, and other industrial chemicals might play a role in delayed puberty.

Diagnosis of Delayed Puberty

- Medical/family history and physical exam in comparison with standard norms
- Blood tests for hormone levels, including levels of gonadotropins (luteinizing hormone, follicle-stimulating hormone) and sex hormones (estrogen, testosterone)
- Bone Age Assessment: A bone age X-ray assesses the individual's skeletal development in comparison to a standard reference.
- Depending on the suspected underlying cause, genetic testing for chromosomal or genetic abnormalities, thyroid function tests, imaging studies, or other specialized tests may be helpful.

Treatment of Delayed Puberty

In many cases, delayed puberty may not require treatment as it can resolve on its own. For instance, the normal age range for the onset of menstruation (menarche) typically occurs between the ages of 9 and 15 years, with most girls experiencing menarche between the ages of 12 and 14. However, it's important to remember that there is a wide range of normal variation, and some girls may start their periods earlier or later than this average range. The term "abnormal" in medicine can mean pathological, but it also can simply mean statistically outside the average range, which can still be healthy. If a girl hasn't started her period by the age of 16 or has other concerns regarding her menstrual development, it's advisable to consult with a healthcare professional, such as a pediatrician or gynecologist, for evaluation and guidance.

If treatment is necessary, the following approaches may be considered:

- **Observation**: For adolescents with constitutional delay of growth and puberty, no specific treatment may be required. Regular monitoring of growth and development is important to ensure that puberty progresses at an appropriate pace.
- **Hormone Therapy**: Hormone therapy may be recommended where there is an identified hormonal deficiency or imbalance. This can involve the use of sex hormones, such as estrogen or testosterone, to initiate and promote puberty.
- **Treatment of Underlying Conditions**: If delayed puberty is caused by an underlying medical condition, such as hypothyroidism or chronic illness, treating the underlying condition may help stimulate puberty.
- **Psychological Support**: Adolescents with delayed puberty may experience emotional and psychological challenges due to the delay in physical development. Providing psychological support, counseling, and education can help them cope with the social and emotional aspects of delayed puberty.
- **Lifestyle Modifications**: In some cases, lifestyle modifications may be recommended to support overall health and development. This can include a balanced diet, regular exercise, and maintaining a healthy weight.

Precocious Puberty

Precocious puberty refers to the early onset of puberty, where sexual and physical maturation occurs earlier than the typical age range. It can have various causes, including:

- **Idiopathic Central Precocious Puberty (ICPP)**: This is the most common cause of precocious puberty. It occurs when the hypothalamus and pituitary gland prematurely activate, causing the early release of hormones responsible for puberty, such as luteinizing hormone (LH) and follicle-stimulating hormone (FSH).

- **Central Precocious Puberty**: This refers to precocious puberty caused by an underlying medical condition affecting the brain, such as a tumor, infection, or injury, which disrupts the normal functioning of the hypothalamus or pituitary gland.
- **Peripheral Precocious Puberty**: In some cases, the early release of sex hormones can be caused by a problem outside the brain, such as a tumor or abnormality in the adrenal glands, ovaries, or testes. This leads to the premature production of estrogen or testosterone, triggering the onset of puberty.
- In **Congenital Adrenal Hyperplasia (CAH)**, decreased cortisol levels result in an increased amount of pituitary ACTH, which can stimulate the adrenal glands to produce excess androgens, causing precocious puberty.
- **Hypothyroidism**: Although usually associated with delayed puberty, long-standing untreated hypothyroidism, particularly in girls, can rarely be associated with precocious puberty (*Van Wyk-Grumbach syndrome*), possibly because elevated levels of thyrotropin-releasing hormone (TRH) might weakly stimulate FSH receptors, leading to premature activation of the reproductive axis. Treatment is through thyroid replacement therapy.
- **Exposure to Hormones**: Certain medications, supplements, or environmental factors can potentially lead to precocious puberty if they contain or mimic sex hormones.
- **Rare Genetic Syndromes**: Certain rare genetic syndromes, such as *Prader-Willi Syndrome*, caused by the deletion of a segment of chromosome 15, can be associated with precocious puberty. *McCune-Albright Syndrome* can cause precocious puberty along with café-au-lait spots on the skin and bone abnormalities. It is caused by a mutation in the GNAS gene.

Diagnosis of Precocious Puberty

The following steps are commonly involved in diagnosing precocious puberty:

- **Medical History**: Gather information about the child's growth, development, and any signs or symptoms of early puberty, as well as the child's family history and any relevant medical conditions.
- **Physical Examination**: Assess the child's growth, pubertal development, and any associated findings. This may include evaluating secondary sexual characteristics, such as breast development in girls or testicular enlargement in boys.
- **Hormonal Evaluation**: Measure the levels of various hormones involved in pubertal development, such as luteinizing hormone (LH), follicle-stimulating hormone (FSH), estrogen, and testosterone.
- **Imaging Studies**: In some cases, X-rays or MRI scans may be recommended to visualize the brain, pituitary gland, or other relevant structures. These imaging tests help identify any structural abnormalities or tumors that may be causing precocious puberty.
- **GnRH Stimulation Test**: This test may be performed to distinguish between central and peripheral precocious puberty. The test involves administering a synthetic GnRH (gonadotropin-releasing hormone) and measuring the response of LH and FSH. In *central precocious puberty*, where the pituitary gland is prematurely sensitive to GnRH, LH and FSH levels should rise, indicating that the hypothalamus-pituitary axis is functioning early. In *peripheral precocious puberty*, where the pituitary gland is typically not prematurely sensitive to GnRH, LH and FSH should not rise.

Treatment of Precocious Puberty

The treatment of precocious puberty aims to slow down or halt the progression of puberty to allow for more normal physical and psychosocial development. The specific treatment approach depends on the underlying cause of precocious puberty and individual patient factors. Treatment may include:

- **Gonadotropin-Releasing Hormone (GnRH) Analog Therapy**: GnRH analogs (e.g., *leuprolide, triptorelin, histrelin, goserelin, nafarelin*) are medications that, when administered in a continuous rather than a normal pulsatile GnRH manner, can suppress the release of gonadotropins (LH and FSH) from the pituitary gland, thereby reducing sex hormone production and slowing down pubertal development. This therapy is the primary treatment for central precocious puberty. GnRH analog therapy can be continued until the appropriate age for puberty to begin.
- **Hormone Blockers**: In some cases, hormone blockers may be used to temporarily halt the effects of sex hormones on pubertal development. These medications, such as anti-androgens (e.g., *spironolactone, flutamide, cyproterone acetate*) or anti-estrogens (e.g., *letrozole, anastrozole,*

exemestane), can be used when there is peripheral precocious puberty.

- **Treatment of Underlying Conditions**: If precocious puberty is caused by an underlying medical condition, such as a tumor, treating it may help manage precocious puberty.

Gynecomastia

Gynecomastia in males can be physiologic or pathologic:

Physiologic gynecomastia occurs with natural fluctuations in hormone levels (androgen/estrogen ratio). About 60-90% of newborns have transient gynecomastia due to circulating estrogen during pregnancy. It usually regresses in 2-3 months after birth.

Pubertal gynecomastia is believed to occur when estrogen levels rise before testosterone levels. It generally regresses within about 18 months and is uncommon after age 17.

Gynecomastia with aging occurs when the testosterone/estrogen ratio decreases, generally between ages 40-80. *Pseudogynecomastia* occurs in obese men and is due to the deposition of fat rather than glandular tissue.

Pathologic gynecomastia can occur with excess estrogen production: estrogen or androgen-secreting testicular or adrenal tumors (testosterone is converted to estrogen), cirrhosis and chronic renal disease (increased conversion of androgens to estrogen), deficient androgen production or androgen insensitivity. Hormone imbalance may be due to drugs that are estrogenic or anti-androgenic. In relatively rare cases, gynecomastia may be due to breast cancer, but that is generally unilateral.

Diagnosis of Gynecomastia

Mild, asymptomatic gynecomastia does not need workup. If it is significant, asymmetric, symptomatic, suspicious for malignancy, or of rapid onset, laboratory tests may include testosterone, estradiol, FHS, LH, TSH, prolactin, and beta-hCG levels (beta-hCG from a secreting tumor can stimulate breast tissue growth). Mammography may be useful if there is a suspicion of malignancy.

Treatment of Gynecomastia

Selective estrogen receptor modulators (e.g., *tamoxifen, raloxifene*) may be used for painful gynecomastia. Testosterone replacement is useful only in hypogonadism. Surgery may be indicated for continued enlargement, tenderness, malignancy, or psychological reasons.

Chapter 18 Infertility

Causes of Infertility

About 15% of married couples have trouble with conceiving. Infertility can be caused by a wide range of factors, both male and female:

Female Causes

1. **Ovulatory disorders**: Problems with ovulation are the most common cause of infertility in women:
    - **Polycystic Ovary Syndrome (PCOS)**: A hormonal imbalance leads to irregular ovulation.
    - **Primary Ovarian Insufficiency (POI)**: A condition where the ovaries stop working normally before the age of 40
    - **Hyperprolactinemia**: Elevated prolactin levels can inhibit ovulation.
    - **Thyroid problems**: Both hyperthyroidism and hypothyroidism can inhibit ovulation.
    - **Tubal blockage**: Scarring from sexually transmitted infections, previous surgeries, or conditions like endometriosis can block the fallopian tubes, preventing sperm from meeting the egg.
    - **Endometriosis**: Endometrial-like tissue outside the uterus can affect the function of the ovaries, uterus, and fallopian tubes.
2. **Uterine or Cervical Abnormalities**:
    - **Uterine fibroids**: Benign tumors in the wall of the uterus
    - **Cervical stenosis**: Narrowing of the cervix
    - **Congenital anomalies**: Birth defects affecting the structure of the uterus and cervix
    - **Early menopause**: Some women experience menopause earlier than the usual age range of late 40s to early 50s.
    - **Pelvic adhesions**: Bands of scar tissue that bind organs after pelvic infection, appendicitis, or abdominal or pelvic surgery
    - **Cervical mucus problems**: Issues with the mucus in the cervix can prevent sperm from traveling up to the fallopian tubes.

Male Causes

- **Varicocele**: Enlargement of the veins in the scrotum can interfere with sperm production.
- **Ejaculation issues**:
    - **Retrograde ejaculation**: Semen enters the bladder during orgasm instead of exiting out through the penis.
    - **Ejaculatory duct obstruction**: Blockage of the ducts from which semen exits
    - **Erectile dysfunction**
- **Anatomical defects of the penis**
- **Tumors**: Cancers and non-malignant tumors can affect the male reproductive organs.
- **Hormonal imbalances**: Disorders of the testicles or pituitary, adrenal or thyroid gland can lead to hormonal imbalances that affect sperm production.

- **Chromosome defects**: Conditions like Klinefelter's syndrome, where a male is born with two X chromosomes and one Y chromosome, can cause infertility.
- **Medications and drugs**: Certain medications (e.g., *sulfasalazine; cimetidine;* anabolic steroids; antihypertensive drugs that cause erectile dysfunction), chemotherapy, radiation treatment, and recreational drugs can reduce sperm production. Excess alcohol and smoking can reduce sperm count and motility.
- **Genetic defects in spermatogenesis**
- **Undescended testicles:** One or both testicles don't descend from the abdomen into the scrotum during fetal development. The higher internal body temperature can impair spermatogenesis.
- **Infections**: Sexually transmitted infections, mumps, or infections of the reproductive organs can affect sperm count and quality.
- **Antibodies** to sperm or seminal fluid

Other Causes and Factors (Both Male and Female)

Unexplained infertility: In a significant number of cases, no cause is found despite investigation.

Age: As age increases, fertility tends to decrease, especially for women after the age of 35. In men, sperm quality generally declines after age 40.

Lifestyle factors: Smoking, excessive alcohol use, drug use, excessive weight (either overweight or underweight), and high stress can contribute to infertility.

Environmental factors: Overexposure to certain environmental factors such as pesticides, radiation, and toxins can decrease fertility.

Cancer treatments: Both radiation and chemotherapy can impair fertility.

Medical conditions: Some medical conditions, like celiac disease, can impact fertility.

Medications: Some medications, including birth control pills, NSAIDs (which can impair prostaglandin synthesis) taken around the time of ovulation, certain antipsychotics and antiepileptic drugs, thyroid medications, some antiretroviral drugs, and antihypertensive drugs that cause erectile dysfunction can affect fertility.

Each individual's or couple's situation is unique, and the cause of infertility can be due to a combination of factors.

Infertility Workup

A fertility workup can vary depending on the medical history and the doctor's experience:

For Females

Medical History and Physical Examination: This includes questions about menstrual cycle regularity, past surgeries, sexually transmitted infections, previous pregnancies, and other relevant health issues. A pelvic exam may also be performed.

Ovulation Testing:

- **Basal Body Temperature Charting**: Tracking daily body temperature to detect the subtle temperature rise that occurs after ovulation
- **Ovulation Predictor Kits**: Home urine tests that detect the surge in luteinizing hormone (LH) that precedes ovulation by about 24 hours
- **Progesterone Blood Test**: Measuring the level of mid-luteal phase progesterone (day 21) in the blood can confirm if ovulation has occurred.
- **Hormonal Evaluation**: Blood tests to check levels of several hormones:
  - FSH (follicle-stimulating hormone)
  - LH (luteinizing hormone)
  - Estradiol
  - Progesterone
  - Prolactin
  - Thyroid hormones (TSH, Free T4)
  - AMH (anti-Müllerian hormone): AMH is a protein produced by the ovarian follicles. Its level provides an index of the number of follicles that have the potential to grow and produce mature eggs in response to fertility treatment.
- **Hysterosalpingogram (HSG)**: An X-ray test that evaluates the shape of the uterus and checks whether the fallopian tubes are open
- **Transvaginal Ultrasound**: To examine the ovaries for cysts or other abnormalities, and to look at the uterine lining
- **Endometrial Biopsy**: A sample of the uterine lining may be taken to check the lining's health and thickness.
- **Laparoscopy** to directly visualize the uterus, fallopian tubes, and ovaries. It can identify endometriosis, scarring, or other tubal or ovarian abnormalities.

For Males:

- **Medical History and Physical Examination**: This includes questions about past surgeries, childhood diseases, medications, sexual history, and other relevant health issues. A physical exam of the testes, penis, and prostate might be performed.
- **Semen Analysis**: The most fundamental test, it evaluates:

- Sperm count (concentration)
- Morphology (shape of the sperm)
- Motility (movement of the sperm)
- Volume of the semen sample
- pH, white blood cell count, and other factors

- **Hormonal Evaluation**: Blood tests to check levels of:
  - Testosterone
  - FSH (follicle-stimulating hormone)
  - LH (luteinizing hormone)
  - Prolactin
- **Testicular Biopsy**: Rarely done, but it can be used if the semen analysis shows very low or no sperm, to determine if the problem is sperm production or sperm transport.
- **Genetic Testing**: To identify any genetic causes of infertility
- **Imaging**: In some cases, imaging tests like an ultrasound might be used to look for testicular, glandular, or structural abnormalities.

The specific tests and their sequence might vary, depending on the individual's or couple's unique circumstances.

Infertility Treatment

Infertility treatments depend on the cause, the duration of infertility, the age of the partners, personal preferences, and other factors:

1. **Medications That Stimulate Ovulation:**
   - **Clomiphene Citrate** *(Clomid, Serophene)* helps stimulate ovulation in women who don't ovulate regularly or who don't ovulate at all. Clomiphene blocks estrogen receptors in the hypothalamus, leading to an increase in the secretion of gonadotropin-releasing hormone (GnRH) from the hypothalamus. The increased secretion of GnRH tricks the pituitary gland into releasing higher levels of follicle-stimulating hormone (FSH) and luteinizing hormone (LH). The increased levels of FSH and LH promote the growth, maturation and release of ovarian follicles (ovulation).
   - **Metformin**: Often used in women with polycystic ovary syndrome to improve insulin sensitivity and promote ovulation
   - **Human Menopausal Gonadotropin** *(Menopur)* or **FSH** *(Gonal-F, Follistim)*: These stimulate the ovaries directly to produce multiple eggs.
   - **Human Chorionic Gonadotropin** *(hCG, Ovidrel, Pregnyl, others)*: Often used in combination with other medications to stimulate the follicle to release the mature egg **Letrozole** *(Femara)*: An aromatase inhibitor used off-label to induce ovulation. It blocks estrogen synthesis. Low estrogen stimulates the pituitary secretion of FSH, which stimulates the ovaries, leading to the growth and maturation of follicles.
   - **Gonadotropin-Releasing Hormone (GnRH) Analogues**: When administered in a continuous rather than a pulsed manner, GnRH analogues control the ovulation process by preventing a premature LH surge that could result in the release of eggs before they can be harvested for in vitro fertilization (IVF). If a GnRH analogue is administered in GnRH's normal pulsatile manner, it *stimulates* the pituitary to release LH and FSH, promoting natural ovulation.
   - **Bromocriptine** *(Parlodel)* **and Cabergoline**: Used for ovulation problems due to excess production of prolactin by the pituitary gland. They suppress prolactin secretion.
2. **Intrauterine Insemination (IUI):** In this procedure, healthy sperm are placed directly in the uterus around the time the ovary releases one or more eggs to be fertilized.
3. **Surgery:** Certain cases of infertility can be corrected or improved with surgical interventions:
   - **Laparoscopic or Hysteroscopic Surgery**: For endometriosis, pelvic adhesions, or certain uterine anomalies
   - **Tubal Surgeries**: To treat blocked or damaged fallopian tubes
   - **Male Surgical Treatments**: For men with obstruction that prevents sperm release, due to injury or infection.
4. **Assisted Reproductive Technology (ART):**
   - **In Vitro Fertilization (IVF)**: The most effective ART, IVF involves retrieving mature eggs from the ovaries, fertilizing them with sperm in a lab, and then implanting the embryos in the uterus.
   - **Intracytoplasmic Sperm Injection (ICSI)**: A single healthy sperm is injected directly into a mature egg during an IVF procedure. This is used when there are significant sperm-related issues.
   - **Gamete Intrafallopian Transfer (GIFT)**: This less commonly used method involves transferring eggs and sperm directly into the fallopian tube, so fertilization can occur naturally inside the body.
   - **Zygote Intrafallopian Transfer (ZIFT)**: Similar to GIFT, but the fertilization of the egg occurs outside the body (as in IVF). Once fertilized, the zygote is then transferred into the fallopian tube.

- **Assisted Hatching**: Helps the embryo to hatch from its protective outer shell and implant in the uterine wall
- **Cryopreservation**: Freezing eggs, sperm, or embryos for future use. This method is useful for those who might lose their fertility due to treatments like chemotherapy or for those who wish to delay childbearing for other reasons.
- **Preimplantation Genetic Diagnosis (PGD) or Screening (PGS)**: Tests embryos for genetic disorders before implantation during an IVF cycle.

5. **Third Party Assistance:**
   - **Egg or Sperm Donation**: Some people choose to use donor eggs or sperm to conceive.
   - **Gestational Carrier (Surrogacy)**: In cases where the woman cannot carry a pregnancy to term, the couple's embryo can be placed in another woman's uterus.
6. **Treatment for Men:**
   Behavioral Changes: Reducing stress, quitting smoking, and limiting alcohol
   Medications: For erectile dysfunction or other hormonal imbalances
   Surgery: To reverse a sperm blockage or repair a varicocele
7. **Other Treatments:**
   Lifestyle Changes: Including weight loss or dietary adjustments.

Chapter 19 Gender Identity Dysphoria

Gender Incongruence refers to the experience of one's gender identity not aligning with their assigned or birth sex, whether or not they experience distress because of the incongruence. People with gender incongruence may describe themselves as *transgender* (*trans*) or *gender diverse*.

Gender dysphoria (formerly called Gender Identity Disorder) is a medical diagnosis used to describe distress or discomfort experienced by individuals whose gender identity differs from the sex assigned to them at birth. People with gender dysphoria may experience significant distress due to a disconnect between their gender identity and their assigned gender.

The term **LGBTQIA+** is an acronym that represents a diverse range of sexual orientations, gender identities, and gender expressions. Each letter in the acronym represents a different group within the broader community:

- **L - Lesbian**: Refers to women who are attracted romantically, emotionally, or sexually to other women.
- **G - Gay**: Refers to men who are attracted romantically, emotionally, or sexually to other men. It is also used as an umbrella term to include all individuals, men or women, who identify as homosexual.
- **B - Bisexual**: Refers to individuals who are attracted romantically, emotionally, or sexually to people of both their own gender and other genders.
- **T - Transgender**: Refers to individuals whose gender identity differs from the sex assigned to them at birth. They may identify as a gender different from the one typically associated with their biological sex. Some surveys suggest that close to 1% of adults in the United States may identify as transgender.
- **Q - Queer** or **Questioning**: "Queer" is an inclusive term that can encompass individuals who have diverse sexual orientations or gender identities that may not fit into traditional categories. "Questioning" refers to individuals who are exploring and questioning their sexual orientation or gender identity.
- **I - Intersex**: Intersex individuals are born with physical sex characteristics (such as chromosomes, hormones, or reproductive anatomy) that do not fit typical definitions of male or female.
- **A - Asexual**: Refers to individuals who experience little or no sexual attraction to others. Asexuality is a spectrum, and individuals may identify as *demisexual* (experiencing sexual attraction after a deep emotional connection is formed) or other related terms. It exists on a continuum.
- **The "+" symbol** represents the inclusion of other sexual orientations, gender identities, and gender expressions that may not be explicitly represented by the letters in the acronym.

The percentage of U.S. adults who identify as LGBT or something other than heterosexual is estimated around 7-8%, an approximate figure influenced by the accuracy of reporting.

It's important to note that the LGBTQIA+ community is diverse, and individuals within these groups may have different experiences, identities, and preferences. The acronym is constantly evolving and may vary in different cultural or regional contexts. It is used as an inclusive term to recognize and respect the diversity of sexual orientations and gender identities beyond the traditional heterosexual and cisgender (where sexual identity aligns with the sex they were assigned at birth) norms.

Most scientists in the field believe that one's sexual orientation likely results from a complex interplay of genetic, hormonal, environmental, and social factors, without a singular cause. There is no established evidence that hormone balance or anatomy differs in homosexual individuals as compared with heterosexuals. There have been some brain studies that raise the question of whether the brains of transgender individuals may align more closely with their gender identity than their sex assigned at birth, but at the time of this writing these studies are inconclusive, as are studies that prenatal hormone exposure might influence gender identity. Hormonal therapy for gender dysphoria is not "correcting an imbalance" but rather bringing one's physical characteristics more in line with their gender identity.

Diagnosis of Gender Dysphoria

The **diagnosis** of gender dysphoria involves a thorough evaluation of a person's gender identity and experiences to determine if they meet the diagnostic criteria outlined in the Diagnostic and Statistical Manual of Mental Disorders (DSM-5):

1. **Assessment of Gender Identity**: The mental health professional conducts interviews and discussions to explore the individual's gender identity, including their feelings, thoughts, and experiences related to their gender. This assessment aims to understand if there is a consistent and persistent identification with a gender different from the one assigned at birth.
2. **Evaluation of Dysphoria**: Assessment of the level of distress or discomfort experienced by the individual due to the incongruence between their gender identity and assigned gender
3. **Review of Symptoms**: The DSM-5 criteria for gender dysphoria include a strong desire to be of a different gender, significant distress or impairment related to their assigned gender, and the persistence of these feelings for a specified duration.
4. **Differential Diagnosis**: The mental health professional will consider other possible explanations for the individual's feelings and experiences to rule out alternative causes. They may explore factors such as cultural or social influences, psychiatric conditions, or other medical conditions that could contribute to the distress.

It is important to note that the diagnosis of gender dysphoria is not about labeling or pathologizing individuals but rather providing a framework for understanding their experiences and accessing appropriate care and support. The diagnosis is used to guide treatment decisions and access to gender-affirming interventions, such as hormone therapy or gender-confirming surgeries, if desired by the individual.

Treatment of Gender Identity Dysphoria

The treatment for gender dysphoria aims to support individuals in aligning their gender identity with their gender expression and achieving improved well-being. The primary approach to treatment is often referred to as *gender-affirming care*, which focuses on affirming and supporting a person's self-identified gender. Some common components of the treatment for gender dysphoria include:

- **Psychotherapy**: Mental health professionals experienced in working with gender diverse individuals can provide individual therapy, group therapy, or family therapy to help individuals explore their gender identity, address any associated distress or concerns, and develop coping strategies. Therapy can provide emotional support, assist with navigating social and familial challenges, and help with decision-making related to transition options.
- **Social Transition**: Social transition involves adopting the gender identity that aligns with a person's self-perception and expressing it in their daily life. This can include using a new name and pronouns, changing gender presentation (clothing, hairstyles, etc.), and coming out to friends, family, and colleagues. Social transition can help alleviate gender dysphoria by allowing individuals to live authentically and be recognized and respected in their affirmed gender.
- **Hormone Therapy**: For individuals seeking to align their physical characteristics with their gender identity, hormone therapy may be an option. Hormone therapy involves the use of hormones, such as testosterone for transgender men or estrogen and anti-androgens for transgender women, to induce physical changes that align with the individual's affirmed gender. Hormone therapy is typically overseen by qualified healthcare professionals and requires ongoing monitoring.

- **Gender-Affirming Surgeries**: Some individuals may opt for gender-affirming surgeries, also known as sex reassignment surgeries, to modify their physical characteristics to align with their gender identity. These surgeries can include procedures such as chest reconstruction (for transgender men), breast augmentation (for transgender women), genital reconstruction surgery, and other procedures that address dysphoric body features. Access to gender-affirming surgeries may vary based on individual circumstances, healthcare systems, and regional regulations.
- **Supportive Care**: Access to support networks, peer support groups, and organizations that provide resources and advocacy for gender diverse individuals can be important in the overall treatment and well-being of individuals with gender dysphoria.

Pros and Cons of Treating Gender Identity Dysphoria

Treating gender dysphoria can have a profound impact on the well-being and quality of life of individuals who experience it. However, it is important to recognize that the perceived pros and cons may vary depending on the individual and their specific circumstances:

Pros of Treating Gender Dysphoria

- **Alleviation of Gender Dysphoria**: Treatment can help alleviate the distress and discomfort associated with the incongruence between a person's gender identity and their assigned sex at birth. By aligning their gender identity with their gender expression, individuals may experience reduced anxiety and depression, and improved mental well-being.
- **Improved Quality of Life**: Treatment can lead to an improved overall quality of life by allowing individuals to live authentically, be recognized and respected in their affirmed gender, and develop a stronger sense of self. This can positively impact self-esteem, self-confidence, and interpersonal relationships.
- **Reduction in Psychological Distress**: Gender-affirming care, including therapy and support, can provide individuals with coping strategies, emotional support, and tools to navigate social and emotional challenges related to their gender identity. This can lead to a reduction in psychological distress and improved psychological well-being.
- **Social Support and Community Connection**: Treatment for gender dysphoria often involves connecting with support networks, peer groups, and organizations that provide resources, validation, and a sense of belonging. Building social support systems and connections with others who share similar experiences can be empowering and provide a sense of community.

Cons of Treating Gender Dysphoria

- **Challenges and Stigma**: Individuals seeking treatment for gender dysphoria may face various challenges, including societal stigma, discrimination, and lack of understanding from others. These challenges can impact mental health and overall well-being.
- **Financial Costs**: Some gender-affirming interventions, such as hormone therapy and surgeries, can be costly. Access to healthcare and insurance coverage for these treatments can vary, and individuals may face financial barriers to accessing care.
- **Risks and Side Effects**: Some medical interventions, such as hormone therapy and surgeries, carry potential risks and side effects. These can include hormone-related changes, surgical complications, implications for fertility, and the need for ongoing medical monitoring.
- **Decision-Making and Individual Choice**: Treatment decisions for gender dysphoria are highly personal and depend on individual preferences, goals, and circumstances. Some individuals may experience uncertainty or difficulty in making decisions related to treatment options and may require time for exploration and self-reflection.
- **Treating gender dysphoria in children** is a complex and evolving topic, which raises some other issues. Currently there is a lack of long-term data on the outcomes of various treatment approaches. There is also the issue of children changing their mind during puberty or after following a course of therapy. While puberty blockers are considered reversible, there is a concern about their long-term effects on physical development and fertility. Surgical changes to the anatomy can be permanent. Treating gender dysphoria in children may involve navigating societal and family acceptance. Some families and communities may struggle to understand or accept the child's gender identity, which can create additional challenges and stress for the child. There is also the issue of obtaining child and parental consent, when this may differ from that of the healthcare provider.

Chapter 20 **Dyslipidemia and Metabolic Syndrome**

Dyslipidemia refers to abnormal blood levels of lipids (such as cholesterol and triglycerides). It is often characterized by elevated LDL cholesterol ("bad" cholesterol; LDL-C) and / or decreased HDL cholesterol ("good" cholesterol; HDL-C), along with increased triglyceride levels. Abnormal levels provided by the American Heart Association and other medical organizations include:

Total Cholesterol – High: 240 mg / dL and above

LDL Cholesterol – High: 160-189 mg / dL and above (< 100 desirable)

HDL Cholesterol – Low (increased risk): < 40 mg / dL for men, < 50 mg / dL for women

Triglycerides – High: 200-499 mg / dL; Very High: 500 mg / dL and above (< 150 normal)

Dyslipidemia is a significant risk factor for cardiovascular diseases, including atherosclerosis and heart disease.

While dyslipidemia is not an endocrine disorder, certain endocrine conditions can contribute to its development. Several endocrine hormones play significant roles in regulating lipoprotein levels and overall lipid metabolism:

Thyroid Hormones: Thyroid hormones impact lipid metabolism. Hypothyroidism is associated with an increase in low-density lipoprotein cholesterol (LDL-C). Hyperthyroidism can lead to reduced LDL-C levels.

Insulin and Insulin Resistance: Insulin affects lipoprotein metabolism. Insulin resistance is often associated with dyslipidemia and can lead to increased levels of triglycerides and reduced levels of HDL-C.

Obesity and Adipokines: Adipose tissue produces hormones known as *adipokines*, which have a variety of physiological functions. In obesity, the balance of these adipokines is altered, leading to changes in lipoprotein metabolism. Obesity is associated with increased levels of triglycerides and decreased levels of HDL-C.

Sex Hormones: Sex hormones, such as estrogen and testosterone, also impact lipid metabolism. Deficiency in estrogen or testosterone has been linked to unfavorable changes in lipoprotein profiles and cardiovascular disease. During menopause, a decline in estrogen production can lead to an increase in LDL-C and a decrease in HDL-C.

Growth Hormone (GH) and Insulin-Like Growth Factor 1 (IGF-1): Growth hormone and IGF-1 also influence lipoprotein metabolism. Growth hormone deficiency can lead to changes in cholesterol and lipoprotein levels that increase the risk for cardiovascular disease.

Cushing's Syndrome: Cushing's syndrome, a condition caused by high levels of cortisol, induces insulin resistance and central adiposity, leading to dyslipidemia, including elevated LDL-C and triglyceride levels and decreased HDL-C.

Of note, dyslipidemia is often multifactorial, resulting from a combination of genetic factors, dietary choices, lifestyle habits, and other underlying medical conditions. Managing dyslipidemia usually involves lifestyle modifications (such as adopting a healthy diet, increasing physical activity, and quitting smoking) along with the administration of medications, like statins to control levels of LDL-C and, to some extent, triglycerides.

Metabolic Syndrome and Obesity

Metabolic syndrome is a cluster of conditions that increase the risk of heart disease, stroke, and diabetes. Metabolic syndrome includes high blood pressure, high blood sugar, excess body fat around the waist, and abnormal cholesterol levels. It may mimic Cushing's syndrome. The syndrome increases a person's risk for heart attack and stroke. Aside from a large waist circumference, most of the disorders associated with metabolic syndrome have no symptoms.

While the exact cause of metabolic syndrome is complex and not completely understood, several factors play a role:

- **Insulin Resistance** leads to elevated glucose levels and over time can lead to type 2 diabetes.
- **Obesity**: Carrying excess weight, especially around the abdomen (central obesity), is a primary risk factor for metabolic syndrome. Studies suggest that genetics contribute to 40-70% of instances of obesity, with over 50 genes involved.
- **Unhealthy Lifestyle**: A sedentary lifestyle, combined with a diet high in unhealthy fats, refined sugars, and processed foods contributes to metabolic syndrome.
- **Hormonal Imbalance**: Insulin resistance, Cushing's syndrome (elevated cortisol), growth hormone disorders (excess or deficiency of growth hormone), hypothyroidism, hyperaldosteronism (hypertension), lipodystrophies, polycystic ovary syndrome, and non-alcoholic fatty liver disease may be associated with metabolic syndrome.
- **Age**: The risk of metabolic syndrome increases with age.
- **Genetics and Family History**: Genetics can increase the risk of metabolic syndrome. If family members have had diabetes, obesity, or metabolic syndrome, the risk may be higher.
- **Race and Ethnicity**: In the United States, Hispanic and non-Hispanic Black populations, compared with non-Hispanic White populations, appear to be at the greatest risk of developing metabolic syndrome.
- **Other Risk Factors**: Smoking, excessive alcohol consumption, and a diet high in carbohydrates can also contribute.

The presence of one or more of the conditions associated with metabolic syndrome increases the risk of serious disease.

Diagnosis of Metabolic Syndrome

A person is diagnosed with Metabolic Syndrome if they have at least three of the following:

Abdominal Obesity (Waist Circumference):
Men: Above 40 inches (102 cm)
Women: Above 35 inches (88 cm)

High Blood Pressure:

- Systolic blood pressure ≥ 130 mm Hg
- Diastolic blood pressure ≥ 85 mmHg

High Fasting Blood Glucose: ≥100 mg/dL
High Triglycerides: ≥ 150 mg/dL
Low HDL Cholesterol:.

- Men: < 40 mg/dL
- Women: < 50 mg/dL

Treatment of Metabolic Syndrome

The treatment for metabolic syndrome involves the management of its individual risk factors, to reduce the overall risk of developing cardiovascular disease, type 2 diabetes, and other metabolic complications. The treatment may involve lifestyle modification and medication.

Lifestyle Modifications

- **Healthy Diet:** Adopt a balanced and heart-healthy diet. Consume whole grains, fruits, vegetables, lean proteins, and healthy fats while limiting added sugars, refined carbohydrates, and saturated and trans fats.
- **Regular Physical Activity:** Engage in regular aerobic exercise, such as walking, jogging, swimming, or cycling, for at least 150 minutes per week. Strength training exercises are also beneficial.
- **Weight Management:** Achieve and maintain a healthy weight through the combination of healthy diet and regular physical activity.
- **Smoking Cessation:** Quite smoking to reduce the risk of cardiovascular disease and other complications.
- **Stress Management:** Manage stress through relaxation techniques, mindfulness, or other stress-reducing activities.
- **Regular Medical Follow-ups:** Monitor progress, adjust treatments, and manage complications.

Medications to manage individual risk factors, such as type 2 diabetes, high blood pressure, and high cholesterol include:

Insulin Resistance and Hyperglycemia:

- **Metformin**: Often the first choice for treating insulin resistance and preventing type 2 diabetes. About 75% of people with type 2 diabetes are obese.
- **Thiazolidinediones** (e.g., *pioglitazone, rosiglitazone*): These can help improve insulin sensitivity but have potential side effects, including weight gain and fluid retention.

Other antidiabetic agents, like SGLT2 inhibitors, GLP-1 agonists, DPP-4 inhibitors, and sulfonylureas, may be used based on individual circumstances and the degree of hyperglycemia.

- ***Hypertension***:
  - **Thiazide diuretics** (e.g., *hydrochlorothiazide*)
  - **ACE inhibitors** (e.g., *lisinopril, ramipril*)
  - **Angiotensin II receptor blockers** (*ARBs;* e.g., *losartan, valsartan*)
  - **Beta-blockers** (e.g., *metoprolol, atenolol*)
  - **Calcium channel blockers** (e.g., *amlodipine, diltiazem*)
  - **Alpha-blockers** (e.g., *doxazosin*)
  - **Renin inhibitors** (e.g., *aliskiren*)
- ***Dyslipidemia***:
  - **Statins** (e.g., *atorvastatin, rosuvastatin, simvastatin*) for reducing LDL cholesterol
  - **Fibrates** (e.g., *fenofibrate, gemfibrozil*): Primarily used to decrease triglyceride levels and may increase HDL cholesterol
  - **Niacin**: Can help to raise HDL cholesterol and lower triglycerides, but its use has declined due to side effects and questionable cardiovascular benefits in the context of newer therapies
  - **Ezetimibe**: Reduces cholesterol absorption from the intestines and can be used alone or in combination with statins
  - **Omega-3 fatty acids**: Can help lower triglyceride levels
  - **PCSK9 inhibitors** (e.g., *evolocumab, alirocumab*): These agents significantly reduce LDL cholesterol. PCSK9 is a protein that binds to LDL receptors, marking them for degradation in the liver. Fewer LDL receptors means less clearance of LDL-C from the bloodstream, leading to increased LDL-C. PCSK9 inhibitors prevent this from happening.
- ***Obesity:*** (see medications below)

Medications for Obesity

Obesity is commonly measured using the **Body Mass Index (BMI)**. The BMI is calculated by dividing an individual's weight in kilograms by their height in meters squared (or [weight in pounds divided by height in inches squared] x 703). A BMI over 25 is considered overweight, and over 30 is obese. High BMI values (typically above 30) are associated with an increased risk of obesity-related health issues.

The major categories of weight loss medications are:

Appetite Suppressants (anorexiants):

Rationale: Appetite suppressants work by targeting the brain's appetite-regulating centers, specifically acting on neurotransmitters like serotonin, norepinephrine, and dopamine. By increasing the levels of these neurotransmitters, they help reduce hunger and increase the feeling of fullness (satiety). This leads to a decrease in food intake and helps with weight loss.

Examples: *phentermine, diethylpropion, phendimetrazine*

Lipase Inhibitors:

Rationale: Lipase inhibitors work by blocking the action of lipase, an enzyme that breaks down dietary fats in the intestines. By inhibiting the absorption of dietary fats, these medications reduce the caloric intake from fats and help promote weight loss.

Example: *orlistat*

GLP-1 Receptor Agonists:

Rationale: GLP-1 (Glucagon-Like Peptide 1) receptor agonists are medications used to treat type 2 diabetes, but they also have weight loss benefits. They work by mimicking the action of GLP-1, a hormone that reduces appetite, slows down gastric emptying, and increases insulin secretion. By activating GLP-1 receptors, these medications help reduce appetite, enhance satiety, and improve glycemic control. *Tirzepatide* (*Zepbound*) is a newer agent that activates both GLP-1 and GIP receptors.

Examples: *liraglutide, semaglutide (Ozempic)*

SGLT-2 Inhibitors:

Rationale: SGLT-2 (Sodium-Glucose Cotransporter-2) inhibitors are primarily used to treat type 2 diabetes. They work by blocking the reabsorption of glucose in the kidneys, leading to increased glucose excretion in the urine. This results in a decrease in blood sugar levels and can also lead to weight loss.

Examples: *canagliflozin, empagliflozin*

Bupropion-Naltrexone Combination:

Rationale: This combination medication works by targeting multiple pathways in the brain. *Bupropion* is an antidepressant that also helps reduce appetite, and *naltrexone* is used to treat opioid and alcohol dependence, but also has appetite-regulating effects.

Together, these medications help reduce food intake and promote weight loss.

It is important to note that weight loss medications are generally prescribed for individuals who are struggling with obesity and who have not achieved sufficient weight loss through lifestyle modifications alone. These medications are most effective when used as part of a comprehensive weight management plan that includes dietary changes, increased physical activity, and behavioral interventions.

Weight Loss Diets

The effectiveness of different diets for weight loss can vary, depending on individual preferences, metabolic factors, and adherence. It's important to find a sustainable and balanced approach that suits the patient's personal needs and promotes overall health:

- **The Low-Fat Diet** focuses on reducing overall fat intake, particularly saturated and trans fats, which raise bad (LDL-C) cholesterol levels, lower good (HDL-C) cholesterol levels, and increase the risk of developing type 2 diabetes. The low-fat diet emphasizes consuming fruits, vegetables, whole grains, lean proteins, and low-fat dairy products. While low-fat diets can be effective for weight loss, they may not be as satiating for some individuals.
- **The Low-Carbohydrate Diet** restricts carbohydrate intake, typically by reducing consumption of refined grains, sugar, and starchy foods. Instead, they emphasize higher protein and fat intake. Low-carbohydrate diets can lead to weight loss and improved blood sugar control, but long-term effects on health are still being studied.
- **The High Protein Diet** emphasizes increased protein intake, which can help reduce appetite and promote muscle growth. Such diets often include lean meats, fish, legumes, and dairy products. High protein diets can support weight loss and muscle maintenance, but it's important to choose lean protein sources and maintain overall dietary balance.
- **The Mediterranean Diet** is rich in fruits, vegetables, whole grains, legumes, lean proteins (such as fish and poultry), and healthy fats (like olive oil and nuts). It emphasizes a balanced and varied approach to eating. The Mediterranean diet has been associated with weight loss, improved heart health, and overall well-being.
- **The Low-Glycemic Diet** focuses on consuming foods that have a lower impact on blood sugar levels, such as whole grains, non-starchy vegetables, and lean proteins. It aims to stabilize blood sugar and insulin levels. While low-glycemic diets may be beneficial for individuals with diabetes or insulin resistance, their impact on weight loss alone is still debated.
- **The Keto Diet** is a high-fat, moderate-protein, low-carbohydrate eating plan. The idea is that ketones from fat breakdown serve as an energy source rather than glucose. Fats include butter, olive oil, coconut oil, avocadoes, nuts, and seeds. Proteins include meat, poultry, fish, seafood, eggs, and cheese. Low-carb veggies include leafy greens, broccoli, cauliflower, zucchini, and bell peppers. The Keto diet avoids bread, rice, pasta, cereals, and sugar. Proponents believe the diet can help with weight loss, while controlling blood sugar.

Ultimately, the best diet for weight loss is one that the person can adhere to long-term and that meets nutritional needs.

Weight Loss Surgery

Restrictive and **malabsorptive procedures** are two types of surgical interventions used for weight loss in individuals with obesity. These procedures aim to reduce the amount of food that can be consumed and/or decrease the absorption of nutrients from the gastrointestinal tract.

- **Restrictive procedures** involve reducing the size of the stomach to limit the amount of food that can be eaten at one time. These procedures create a smaller stomach pouch, which leads to a feeling of fullness with smaller portions of food. Some common restrictive procedures include:
  - *Adjustable Gastric Banding*: A band is placed around the upper part of the stomach, creating a small pouch above it. The band can be tightened or loosened to control the rate of food passage.
  - *Vertical Sleeve Gastrectomy (VSG)*: A portion of the stomach is surgically removed, leaving a smaller sleeve-shaped stomach. This reduces the stomach's capacity and restricts food intake.
  - An *intragastric balloon* may be placed endoscopically to reduce gastric capacity.
- ***Malabsorptive Procedures*** involve rerouting or bypassing a portion of the small intestine, reducing the absorption of nutrients and calories from food. These procedures alter the normal digestive process. Some common malabsorptive procedures include:
  - *Roux-en-Y Gastric Bypass (RYGB):* involves creating a small stomach pouch and connecting

it directly to the middle part of the small intestine. This bypasses a portion of the stomach and small intestine, limiting both food intake and nutrient absorption.

- *Biliopancreatic Diversion with Duodenal Switch (BPD-DS)*: This procedure involves a sleeve gastrectomy to create a smaller stomach, followed by rerouting the intestines to decrease the absorption of nutrients.
- A *gastric emptying system (AspireAssist)* involves placement of a percutaneous gastrostomy tube that connects to a skin port. About one-third of an ingested meal is removed through the port. The procedure is reserved for people unable to achieve weight loss by non-surgical therapy.

Weight loss surgeries are typically considered for individuals with a body mass index (BMI) above a certain threshold and who have not achieved significant weight loss through other methods.

These procedures are often accompanied by comprehensive lifestyle changes, including dietary modifications, increased physical activity, and long-term follow-up care to support successful weight management and overall health.

Index

U

V

W

RAPID LEARNING AND RETENTION THROUGH THE MEDMASTER SERIES:

BASIC SCIENCES:
CLINICAL NEUROANATOMY MADE RIDICULOUSLY SIMPLE, by S. Goldberg
CLINICAL BIOCHEMISTRY MADE RIDICULOUSLY SIMPLE, by S. Goldberg
ORGANIC CHEMISTRY MADE RIDICULOUSLY SIMPLE, by G.A. Davis
CLINICAL ANATOMY MADE RIDICULOUSLY SIMPLE, by S. Goldberg and H. Ouellette
CLINICAL PHYSIOLOGY MADE RIDICULOUSLY SIMPLE, by S. Goldberg
CLINICAL MICROBIOLOGY MADE RIDICULOUSLY SIMPLE, by M.T. Gladwin, B. Trattler and C.S. Mahan
CLINICAL PHARMACOLOGY MADE RIDICULOUSLY SIMPLE, by J.M. Olson
ACID-BASE, FLUIDS, AND ELECTROLYTES MADE RIDICULOUSLY SIMPLE, by R. Preston
PATHOLOGY MADE RIDICULOUSLY SIMPLE, by A. Zaher
CLINICAL PATHOPHYSIOLOGY MADE RIDICULOUSLY SIMPLE, by A. Berkowitz
CLINICAL BIOSTATISTICS AND EPIDEMIOLOGY MADE RIDICULOUSLY SIMPLE, by A. Weaver and S. Goldberg
CONSCIOUSNESS MADE RIDICULOUSLY SIMPLE: A SERIOUS RESOLUTION OF THE MIND/BODY PROBLEM, by S. Goldberg
IS THE MIND IMMORTAL? THE ORIGIN OF CONSCIOUSNESS, by S. Goldberg
CLINICAL GENETICS MADE RIDICULOUSLY SIMPLE, by S. Goldberg

CLINICAL SCIENCES:
OPHTHALMOLOGY MADE RIDICULOUSLY SIMPLE, by S. Goldberg and W. Trattler
PSYCHIATRY MADE RIDICULOUSLY SIMPLE, by J. Nelson, W. Good and M. Ascher
CLINICAL PSYCHOPHARMACOLOGY MADE RIDICULOUSLY SIMPLE, by J. Preston and J. Johnson
BEHAVIORAL MEDICINE MADE RIDICULOUSLY SIMPLE, by F. Seitz and J. Carr
THE FOUR-MINUTE NEUROLOGIC EXAM, by S. Goldberg
CLINICAL RADIOLOGY MADE RIDICULOUSLY SIMPLE, by H. Ouellette and P. Tetreault
THE PRACTITIONER'S POCKET PAL: ULTRA RAPID MEDICAL REFERENCE, by J. Hancock
CLINICAL CARDIOLOGY MADE RIDICULOUSLY SIMPLE, by M.A. Chizner
CARDIAC DRUGS MADE RIDICULOUSLY SIMPLE, by M.A. Chizner and R.E. Chizner
CARDIAC PHYSICAL EXAM MADE RIDICULOUSLY SIMPLE, by M.A. Chizner
ECG INTERPRETATION MADE RIDICULOUSLY SIMPLE, by M.A. Chizner
ORTHOPEDICS MADE RIDICULOUSLY SIMPLE, by P. Tétreault and H. Ouellette
IMMUNOLOGY MADE RIDICULOUSLY SIMPLE, by M. Mahmoudi
ALLERGY AND ASTHMA MADE RIDICULOUSLY SIMPLE, by M. Mahmoudi
RHEUMATOLOGY MADE RIDICULOUSLY SIMPLE, by A.J. Brown
CRITICAL CARE AND HOSPITALIST MEDICINE MADE RIDICULOUSLY SIMPLE, by M. Donahoe and M.T. Gladwin
CLINICAL HEMATOLOGY MADE RIDICULOUSLY SIMPLE, by S. Goldberg
ARE YOU AFRAID OF SNAKES?: A Doctor's Exploration of Alternative Medicine, by C.S. Mahan
WAR AGAINST THE GERMS: EPIDEMICS, MICROORGANISMS, AND BIOWARFARE, by S. Goldberg
ENDOCRINOLOGY MADE RIDICULOUSLY SIMPLE, by S. Goldberg
GASTROENTEROLOGY MADE RIDICULOUSLY SIMPLE, by S. Goldberg and H. Baikovitz
NEUROLOGY MADE RIDICULOUSLY SIMPLE, by S. Goldberg
INTERPRETING MEDICAL LAB SCREENING TESTS MADE RIDICULOUSLY SIMPLE, by S. Goldberg

BOARD REVIEW:
USMLE STEP 1 MADE RIDICULOUSLY SIMPLE, by A. Carl
USMLE STEP 2 MADE RIDICULOUSLY SIMPLE, by A. Carl
USMLE STEP 3 MADE RIDICULOUSLY SIMPLE, by A. Carl
NCLEX-RN MADE RIDICULOUSLY SIMPLE, by A. Carl

OTHER:
MEDICAL SPANISH MADE RIDICULOUSLY SIMPLE, by T. Espinoza-Abrams
MED SCHOOL MADE RIDICULOUSLY SIMPLE, by S. Goldberg
MED'TOONS (260 humorous medical cartoons by the author) by S. Goldberg
THE STUTTERER'S APPRENTICE, by A. Splaver

For further information, see www.medmaster.net or Email: info@medmaster.net.